One Good Woman Come and Gone

A LOVE STORY

By Robert L. Gamble

CHICAGO SPECTRUM PRESS
Louisville, Kentucky

CHICAGO SPECTRUM PRESS
4824 Brownsboro Center
Louisville, Kentucky 40207
800-594-5190

ISBN 1-58374-014-7

Printed in the U.S.A.

10 9 8 7 6 5 4 3 2

7-27-07

For My Loving Wife
Cynthia H. Gamble
1949 – 1993

To Technicolor Days
1975 – 1993

The Joy she gave me has come & gone but Love never Leaves... And I Just want to thank her

Robert L. Gamble

Table of Contents

Introduction

I met my wife Cynthia in October 1975. Both of us were recent divorcees and single parents. It wasn't love at first sight but a relationship that moved steadily in a gradual progression.

She was a date, a plaything, a girlfriend, my woman, a soulmate, and a wife. From the night that we met, it took about six months to confess our love for each other. We became soulmates in a little less than three years, and we became husband and wife in August 1992.

Cynthia died from lung cancer in December 1993, after a gallant ten-month battle. I started writing about our life together two days after she passed because I felt this great need to tell our story. I felt as though writing about us would keep our relationship alive, or keep her alive in my memory. I didn't know that I couldn't forget her, even if I tried. Writing about us was therapeutic to me because it allowed me, in the worst of times, to focus on the best of times.

This book consists of excerpts from a longer journal. I know that being born and dying are incidentals of living, and living and dying are filled with acts of love. So my emphasis is about a love affair, as opposed to a dying affair. Still, I start with dying, the immediate catalyst, as briefly as I can tell it. I saturate my remembrances in rhymes and sketches of our love affair. Today I call all of the loving times we spent together "technicolor days."

My journal is meant to be a celebration of Cyn and me. There are those who can write about a love affair in a clinical manner, those who can follow the suggestion of the television detective who wanted "Just the facts." I'm not one of those people; my journal is vintage me. I would say that I'm loving and thoughtful, but I am also grassroots, narcissistic, comedic, and opinionated. I can't write any other way.

More than anything else, I want my story to be what our technicolor days together really were… a romantic comedy.

The first section is "Technicolor Days: Reflections of Love and Joy." Starting with the day we met, I want the reader to get to know us. The middle sections, "Me and Her: Remembrances of Nights When We Were Happy" and "Melodies: From a Wind Chorus in January," are the backbone of my personal journal. I would have loved to have lingered here longer because these moments are about loving and living. I don't intend to make any concessions to readers who knew what my book was about and they wanted me to "get on" with the dying. Some people have a fascination with sickness, dying, and death. It's a dramatic part of life that some enjoy reading about, as though it is a unique and pleasant experience.

The next section, "Joy: Spirit on the Loose," is about Cynthia's growing spirituality and the spirituality that brought us to the altar. "A Captive in the Camp of Grief and Sadness" is a small glimpse of my ordeal after the loss of the love of my life. "The Sun Setting, Body Storm Rising" is about the ten months of Cyn's illness. It's all about love too; it's the one who is left behind — the last great act of love. I'm hoping that I'll teach my readers something about the importance and the power of love.

Ode: On the Loss of a Good Woman

She was elegant, beautiful
sensual, feline, and delicate
    yet strong
independent, funny, and exciting.

    There might
be unchanging truths about death:
"The sun will still rise in
    the morning and life goes on."

    The truth of
the wedding vows are prophetic:
"In sickness and in health and
    till death do us part."

    And there's
always truth in the Good Book:
"For everything there is a season
a time to be born and a time to die."

    Deep in my soul
I believe she's in Paradise, Heaven

    but when I'm alone
    in a dark empty house
    in a cold lonely bed
    in the black early morning
    I'm consumed by only one truth,
    my pretty woman is gone.
And she won't be coming home anymore.

Reverberating

If you really understand me
you are deeply in love,
        or
you've been deeply in love and
you know the splendor and the joy.

        If
you're feeling what I'm feeling
you've been deeply in love
suddenly lost that love and
you know my pain and my sorrow,

        but please
don't pause on loving and losing
if you can help it,
count your blessings and let
life, loving, and joy consume you.

        One way
or another it will all end, but
riding the currents of the wind,

        reverberating
around the Earth forever are
the echoes of voices of lovers,
like yours, like hers and mine

        still whispering
"I love you… I love you too."

It's Gone, Gone, Gone

When you cross the River Jordan
    they say
you can't take it with you, but
    they lied.
They don't know, they don't love
the way I do because she did and
    it's gone, gone, gone...

Chased her, love stopped running
grabbed my hand, wouldn't let go
    I'm captured
joy exploded, blessings gushed
but they left with her and they're
    gone, gone, gone...

    A hug
one and only like a fingerprint
her face is pressed on my chest
    I'm drinking
her scent and the scent of her
soft, aromatic hair, but they're
    gone, gone, gone...

I'm just not who I used to be.

Can't laugh as heartily anymore
although they don't say anything
    I know
they can hear the rattlings from
    my empty insides
yet they still believe you can't
take it with you but she did and
    it's gone, gone, gone.

Close to Midnight: 12-22-1993

The battle was over… She was gone forever… I was alone. As empty as I felt, as bone-tired, it would seem that I would just collapse on the bed, with my clothes still on, in a long, deep sleep. It was not to be; my bad luck continued. I was lying there feeling that strange feeling of sadness intertwined with relief. It was Wednesday, and she had been placed on a respirator the previous Wednesday. The respirator had broken my will. I had cried to the God that raised Lazarus to save her or carry her to paradise.

That night I thought about that day just ten months ago. I was home alone when Cyn called saying that dreadful word *cancer*. After I hung up the phone, I remember just crying and saying over and over, "It ain't fair!" I met her at her mother's house. I was able to contain my crying for a while on my way to the apartment, and I was shocked to see that she hadn't shed a single tear. I didn't want to cry in front of her, especially since she was not crying. I waited in the apartment while she took the elevator up to her cousin's apartment to give her the bad news. I talked to her mother, who wasn't crying either, but I had started crying again. It occurred to me that these ladies were bearing up, and I was falling apart. It was Cynthia and her mother's faith and spirituality that was giving them the strength I needed but did not have.

We went for a walk when Cynthia returned. She told me she wasn't afraid of dying; she just didn't want to suffer. It was Wednesday, and that night we attended an intercessory prayer meeting at Cynthia's church, the Apostolic Church of God. It was a joyous meeting of praying, singing, and clapping to music. Practically everybody was standing but me. I was sitting there unable to stop my tears from flowing when Cynthia motioned me to stand. After singing and swaying to the music for a while, she turned to me and whispered in my ear, "I'm going to live with Jesus."

On the sad night Cynthia passed over to God, I was experiencing a lot of conflicting feelings, and I had become more angry than anything else. I was steaming mad because it just felt right. It seemed to have put something in my stomach, and it felt better being boiling mad than being empty. I was thinking, "To hell with everything. My woman is gone. The love of my life is dead." The word "dead" is worse than hearing the word "cancer." I prefer to hear "passed," "gone," or "crossed the river." But whatever it's called, she's not coming back, and it just ain't fair. Murderers, junkies, rapists, and criminals were still alive, and many live into their sixties and eighties. Cynthia was a good mother, wife, humanitarian, Christian, and an asset to the world. Does being innocent, good, or "saved" get you anywhere? Will the meek really inherit the Earth?

Cynthia's mother was grieving very hard that terrible night. She told me that the old wives tale of nothing being harder on a mother than the loss of a child is true. Throughout Cyn's illness she would say, "I can't give her up." But even during those times, she maintained a Christian outlook, saying, "All souls belong to Him." On the other hand, I was wallowing in self-pity and thinking that there was no man sadder than a one-woman man whose woman had died. I thought about men who have more than one woman, a bachelor with several girlfriends, and men with wives and women on the side. I kept thinking that I had one woman, whom the sun rose and set with, and I had lost her.

For the next few days, I prayed more than I ever had, desperately trying to close some kind of a spiritual gap that would give me some peace. Still, I couldn't be peaceful and accepting. I was trying, but I just couldn't envision my Cynthia in heaven. I was envisioning a frail, broken body lying in a cold storage on 79th Street in Chicago. I was not mad at God. I'm a believer, and I was afraid to be mad at my creator. Like others, and especially at this time, I was unable to understand and accept His will without question. Either way, Cynthia's problems were over, and my problems had really just started. I was mad at life's unfairness, and I was overwhelmed by those feelings.

We had prayed over and over for the miracle of Cyn's health being restored. It didn't happen, but I still had not given up on a miracle. On that sad Wednesday night, I was wishing to see her spirit. I wanted to see Cyn whole once more. I've heard all of my life that things like this can happen. I was hoping she would appear in a vision, and that she would be smiling that pretty smile I had not seen for ten months. On that day of her biopsy, the radiant sparkle in her eyes was replaced by a sadness; a sadness that would deepen and never leave.

If Cyn had appeared, I wanted her to tell me that she was at peace, out of pain, in a better place, and for me not to be sad. I wanted to hear her say that I had done all right, that I had made the right decisions during the battle. I kept thinking about how we had only focused on her getting well, and so many other things were left unsaid. I felt this great need to hear many things that were unspoken, even at this late hour.

For months I had the feeling that the inside of a car was the last private place I would find in America. It was my crying room; a place where I didn't have to look stoic or appear to be strong. I felt I needed to appear this way in front of

Cynthia. When I was with her, I had to be positive and show that I had absolute faith that everything was going to turn out all right. I wasn't just pretending; part of me really had faith that everything would turn out all right. I put the notion that some are saved and some are not in the back of my mind. And why shouldn't my wife, a good servant of the Lord, be in that number that was to be saved? I just knew that she would go into complete remission or at least survive for no less than five years. I was thinking that under the circumstances, this would be enough time for us to be happy and really appreciate every single day. It would also give us enough time to prepare for the inevitable in life.

Unable to sleep in the blackness of the early dawn, I decided to drive along Lake Shore Drive seeking the truth of the quote, "The sun will still rise in the morning and life goes on." We had taken this drive many times. Cyn and I loved the lake and Lake Shore Drive, because it's such a pretty place to drive along. In the summer, the bright sun shone on her soft hair, almond-brown face, and sculptured lips. Gentle Lake Michigan breezes filled the air with the scent of her sensual perfume, and just my being with my sweet baby filled me with joy and love.

In summer, bikers and joggers jockeyed for space on the trail, winding its way beside Lake Michigan. On the beach, a mother held her toddler while he splashed his tiny feet in the warm shallow waters. But that was then; it was no longer summertime. It was the worst of times for me — a freezing December 23, 1993. The morning after the day my wife Cynthia crossed the River Jordan.

Sunrise on a Grim Reaper's Dawn

in wintertime
in cryingtime
flowers don't drink from crystal
but lie shivering atop
brushed-steel, cold gravestones
and the
first faint light of dawn brings
no summer sounds, morning sounds,

I drove slowly
in half-darkness beside a stilled
Great Lake stripped-naked of all
that once held me together but I
needed to know, "Will
the sun still rise in the morning?"

sooty-snow piled along the Drive
gave way to pure white drifts far
into the lake,
row after row of snow waves were
immobile, unstirring, arctic-like
near the shore
scattered blocks of ice protruded
ice-fragments resembled
colossal pieces of shattered glass,

vapor, ghost-like, rose
off the lake, maybe December mist
off icy-waters or was
it smoke from a muted burning sun
pushing its head from the depths
of a watery grave

childish-like the sun's forehead
peeked over a distant range of
stunning plum-purple mountains,
    alas, they were
darken-clouds asleep at the foot
    of the lake's horizon

    the eastern sky
a dimness creeping into daylight
    became a fusion
of lavender, tangerine, sky-blue
    on the beach
billions of suns flickered in
pretty crystalline ice-fragments
    dispersed sowed-like,

    grabbing sunglasses
I intended to look in the eyes of
the rising sun, hoping it'll dry
the moisture I couldn't stop from
    swelling in my eyes,

lingering surrealistically time
    seemed suspended

    I was drawn to
our nearest star as never before,
completely ignoring common sense
what every child's been taught
never look directly at the sun

but I was transfixed,
trying, but couldn't turn away
I know what's real
what's not real but
unfamiliar, unexplored feelings
conceptualized that
something powerful, very unusual
was inescapable

I welcomed the strange feelings
sensing no danger
I sensed this a defining moment
although thinking, but for what?

instantly
the hum of my car's engine went
totally silent
a hush unknown to me had joined
the Grim Reaper's dawn, joyless
enough without
summer sounds or morning sounds

believably
unbelievably
I began hearing roarings of the
sun burning,
sounds louder than forest fires
out of control
galloping thru dry-canyons in
a hot, rainless California summer

paranormal, bewailing,
extra-sensory perception?
is deep-grief hypnotic, psychotic

and unrelated questions
flooded my mind but I had no time
to reflect for without
time passing I saw flames flaring
off the sun's surface

reddish-orange
yellow, purple, lavender-blue but
I couldn't accept it unwaveringly,
had I been drugged by
grief, surely as if it was opium?

like a molten river
a long trail of gases shot from the
base of the sun and it resembled
a nonchalant comet rising from the
bowels of the Earth,

suddenly, as
quickly as it had risen straight
the sun veered like an asteroid
falling
burning, whining, heading to crash,

am I dreaming about the dead, or
am I the dead dreaming I'm alive?

halting, the sun wasn't rising or
    falling but without
time passing the sun headed-down,
its gaseous tail wagged like the
tail of a kite that's snapped its
string and zig-zags toward tall
    distant treetops

        soon, as if the
thermal fires had been smothered,
    the roaring stopped,
total-silence as the sun floated,
    astounding, awesome
    wonderful, beautiful

it dived into far horizon-waters,
a deafening thud, a steam cloud
rose as a dull-orange spheroid
like the vanishing, upturned-bow
    of the Titanic slid
hissing into a mammoth sink-hole,

the sun had answered my question
    it had bowed its
head on my first day of grieving,

the love of my life is gone but
on a Grim Reaper's dawn, maybe
only in my head, on an illusory
Great Plains of roses and orchids
where wistfulness slays reality,
    the sun didn't
just… still rise in the morning.

To everything there is a season,
A time for every purpose
under heaven:
A time to be born,
And a time to die…[3:2]
A time to weep
And a time to laugh.[3:4]

– *ECCLESIASTES* 3:2 & 3:4

TECHNICOLOR DAYS: REFLECTIONS OF LOVE AND JOY

Technicolor Days

A
time of death isn't always requiem
dark, somber,
purple and black
or processional with muffled drums
riderless horses
horsedrawn carriages.

A time of death is also happy days
harvest time,
crisp, sunny days
splashed with pastel colors, like

the technicolor days of autumn.

While
they were alive they were green,
now colorful carcasses of leaves
oblong, linear, elliptic, deltoid
all float by.

They're
burnt-orange, brown, golden, plum,
sienna, saffron, olive, and crimson,

splashin' and struttin'
in and around ponds, lagoons are
wood ducks in colorful iridescent
greens
purples
blues and
gray mallards with chestnut breasts.

Retreating overhead
are waterfowl in a V formation,
Canada geese,
brownish body, a long black neck,
a white patch on the cheek;
wave after wave
flying in cold, clear-blue skies
honking, screaming,
heading south looking for places
where dog days linger.

Metamorphic autumn,
the last rites for long hot days
and in this
time of passing summer radiance
clings to life,

spectacular colorful blooms,

purple and white morning glories
giant sunflowers, pink begonias
red roses, lavender periwinkles,
all will languish before falling

Green will fade but not disappear.

Retreating daylight,
like a boychild will run home to
the west earlier every evening,
like a shadow, duskiness follows
and
apologetic for leaving early the
evening sky will dress in patchy
wispy-pretty altostratus sunsets.

In the parks,
brownish-gray stone bridges curl
gracefully across murky lagoons.

The Great Lake,
sometimes blue, sometimes green,
sometimes greenish-blue.

In the Loop,
skyscrapers, terra cotta, glass
metallic, old and new brick.

In Midwestern fields,
in broad, picturesque orchards
tiny seeds have sprouted plump
orange pumpkins, round and heavy,
and
maize-colored corn lies in deep
furrows below green and flaxen
towering stalks.

Scarecrows
in yesterday's high fashions,
garish-colored and mismatched
are tall, indifferent, silent
and intimidating

Against a turquoise autumn sky.

Wintertime,
misty, pearl-gray and snow-white
must stand in waiting, for the
Earth's ornamented itself with
the technicolor days of autumn.

First Meeting: Another Pretty Face

In autumn, there's a beauty about Chicago that's a harmony of man-made things and nature. This is especially evident when you live near the lake, and if you drive up and down Lake Shore Drive often. The lake is your playground: you can picnic, bike, jog, sail, or just walk along the lake, and you'll fall in love with its beauty. I really love a beautiful day. I used to tell Cynthia that I really felt spiritual on a spectacular, beautiful day. On one of those days I would say, "Baby, today is a technicolor day."

I used the expression "technicolor days" in reference to a joyful time in my youth. When I was a preteen and a teenager, my friends and I attended a lot of movies. Those movies were made in the thirties, forties, and fifties, and many of them were made in black and white. Certain movies were made and advertised as being in technicolor, and that alone was enough to get us to go see it. We were young, and we weren't into any art nouveau appreciation of black and white films. We thought that technicolor was beautiful and natural. All of the days I spent with Cynthia... I see as the most beautiful days of my life, and I love to call them "technicolor days."

In 1985 Cynthia and I had our ten-year anniversary as soulmates. I remember saying, "Ten long years! I just wanted a one-night stand. How in the hell did you manage to stretch it out this long?"

She said, "I felt sorry for you. I didn't want your family

coming after me because you slashed your wrist when I gave you your walking papers."

That was a typical exchange between us. We were both jive-talking, fun people; our long relationship wasn't stormy, but full of jokes and laughter. We joked a lot about the first impressions we had of each other on the evening we first met. I was always amazed at how we could recall so many of the things the other said in that first meeting. As a history teacher, I was always teaching about the various factors that lead to certain events, so without thinking, I was always analyzing and overanalyzing my social life. Looking back, I think it was two social trends of the mid-seventies that brought us together.

By the mid-seventies, a practice that had been sort of frowned upon years earlier was well-established in Chicago. I'm speaking of the practice of women, in general, going into a bar without a male escort. Women were working jobs in fields they were not allowed in before. They had taken up one of their male co-workers favorite habits, which was stopping at a bar before going home, for what was generally known as an after-work drink. There were many women in groups with girlfriends and other co-workers, males and females. Women had broken down another of the many double-standard rules imposed upon them in our society. For bachelors, this new trend was a great step forward. It meant more educated, professional, career-minded, working women were now on the social dating scene. Not only were they out there in numbers, but they had money, and buying their own drinks was no big thing.

Another trend prevalent in the early seventies, one of which I was a part, was a wave of divorces sweeping the country. I had been divorced in 1974, and it seems as though half of the women I met were either divorced or in the process of getting one. The opening up of fields once closed to women and their growing economic power brought about many new freedoms for them. Not only could they buy their own drinks, but they also had the ability to support themselves and leave their bad marriages.

Cynthia was in that number of women divorced in 1975, but we didn't meet on Lonely Avenue. Both of our lives were in an upswing; we were both sifting through dates and offerings of dates. I met Cynthia on a technicolor day in October 1975. It was a late Friday evening after a football game played by the high school where I taught history, Englewood High School. Usually after a game a number of faculty members and coaches would meet at a prearranged lounge for a victory celebration. A group of us bachelors had found this great lounge on east 75th Street in South Shore. It was a perfect meeting place for the after-work set. People that lived in the South Shore area would ride the Illinois Central Metra train to and from work in the Loop, and one of its stops was on 75th Street and Exchange. This is where I met Cynthia with a bunch of her girlfriends one Friday evening after a game.

The barstools that evening were lined with good-looking women; a lot of co-workers and girlfriends were there without male escorts. I specifically recall that there were several politicians in the bar that day, including the ward alderman. The ward office was about a half block away. This lounge was also frequented by many off-duty police officers, and then there was my faculty group. Most teacher groups were well known by the bartenders because we got off work the earliest and we were usually the first after-work group to arrive and to leave. During the week, if we came and stayed for a couple of hours, we could be gone before the nine-to-five crowd got off work.

Cynthia and her girlfriends Carol, Joann, and Gloria were together. I only knew Carol. Probably by coincidence, they were mostly light-skinned beauties, but I was drawn to Cynthia, an almond-brown skinned woman. I told her later in the relationship that it was nothing more than simply being attracted to a pretty face. I always like to observe faces because I believe I'm able to read them and quickly get a feeling of the persona. I thought I could judge a woman's happiness, loneliness, and whether she had led a hard or soft life through her eyes. I was not always right, but when I could add an hour of conversation to my initial facial impression, I was very seldom completely off-base.

The expression "looking at the world through rose-colored glasses" denotes that a person is seeing things not as they really are. But there are stretches in a person's life when life is joyful, rose-colored, and somehow the person knows that the best is yet to come. That was the time in my life when I met Cynthia. The autumn day I met her was crisp, clear, and technicolor. The night was also crisp, clear, and very dark, but that was outside. Inside my favorite lounge, it was vintage south-side Chicago nightlife. The lounge was full of soulful music, getting-down music, and slow-dancing music. The place was packed. Some were looking for love, and some were looking for lust.

I fought my way through the crowded lounge feeling like I was moving in slow motion. There was a myriad of stunning colored girls under a myriad of colorful lights. I believe that everything that's pretty comes in colors. Pretty man-made things like paintings, lipstick, and lace lingerie. In nature, there are sunsets, butterflies, and wildflowers. So it stands to reason that the sisters would come in many beautiful colors. They're almond, fawn, ebony, tan, hi-yellow, chocolate, olive, redbone, and sepia.

As I moved slowly around, I felt as if I were in a dreamland of pleasant scents and colors. It was like being a boy again on Christmas morning looking at all of those colorful wrapped presents under the tree. Tonight, it's the lights, dresses, jeans, corporate suits with silk blouses, jewelry, lip stick, and different colors of hair. But it was skin, the colored flesh, that sustained my fascination. The various hues of all of those colored girls sensually assaulted my senses. Those cute faces, bare shoulders and backs, full cleavages, and long, pretty legs, crossed and dangling from tall barstools.

I kept moving and looking over the rainbow beauties lining the bar, glancing, but not staring. A bashfulness that has followed me from childhood just wouldn't allow me to lock eyes with a pretty lady. So I moved and glanced around for a while before my eyes landed right on Cynthia. Her face was heart-shaped and almond; her hair was reddish, sort of long and soft looking. She kept laughing with her friends about something, and as she did her teeth flashed and her eyes sparkled. Being bashful, I didn't look directly at her. Fortunately, I could see her clearly in the mirror, so I stared a while at the pretty woman laughing. She looked classy and very sophisticated, but her lips were tribal and primitive. I was thinking, "Damn! that's one pretty black thing." I noticed that she had no ring on her finger. Still, I figured she probably had somebody, but he was nowhere around, so I could go ahead and make my move. I was wondering how she would react to the shortest line in my repertoire. I would walk up to her, get her attention, and say, "Woman… you need me!" Then I would walk off, let it sink in, and get back to her at a later time.

I slid onto the barstool beside Cynthia as soon as I got a chance, and I struck up a friendly conversation. It turned out to be one of those, "Isn't it a small world," conversations. I soon learned that she had graduated from Englewood High School. In fact, I started working there her senior year, but we didn't know one another. I was sort of disappointed that she was a student in the same building for a whole year, and she had never heard my name. But upon reflection, it was my first year, and I hadn't made my mark around the school. Anyway, this coincidence gave her the opportunity to sit and praise some of the teachers and to dog a few others. Overall, she was sort of proud of her high school, especially the friends she had made while attending. I asked her if she was intimidated by sitting in a bar talking to one of her "old teachers." She said, "No, my mother's an old teacher."

A couple of years later, she said when we first started talking she thought that we were roughly around the same age, and she was surprised to find out that I was ten years older than she. This didn't surprise me since I had always looked younger than my age, and I told her that if I thought she was my same age, I wouldn't have wasted my time talking to her. I was joking. I really wasn't hung up on a woman's age.

I was more friendly than aggressive, and I think that strategy paid off. Maybe it was her girlfriend, Carol, that gave me the stamp of approval, because before Cyn's group left that night, she invited me to come and play cards with them sometime. I said I would, but a card party wasn't my idea of a good time. I didn't play well, and I knew black people take bid whist very seriously. If you couldn't play well, your best bet was not to even sit down, and I could tell they were serious players. Years later, Cyn told me that she was surprised I didn't ask for her phone number that first night. I knew I would see the group again, and asking for phone numbers right away was just not my style. Hell, I wanted to know why she didn't ask for mine!

I believe most women are somewhat intuitive, and they think they can size men up in a glance. I always believed a woman's first impression of me was the big brother type of guy. Some women used to tell me that I was the friendly, marrying kind, not the type of man that hits on every skirt. They were half-way right. I wasn't really the marrying kind especially after a divorce, but I am overtly friendly, joking, and brotherly because I have always accepted women as friends, as well as being colleagues.

The next time I saw Cynthia, she was standing with her little girl at a counter in a Kentucky Fried Chicken restaurant. I saw her in the bright, non-lounge lights for the first time. I was thinking that her true beauty shone. Her daughter was a carbon copy of her in miniature, and they stood there holding hands. The sight of them touched me in that wonderful primal, paternalistic sense of aesthetics.

I asked, "Who is this pretty little girl?" She introduced us. I remembered that she was divorced, and I wasn't about to let her just disappear again. I had a policy of not asking for a woman's phone number, but I readily gave her mine. This was to let her know that I wasn't married, and also it saved me from possibly being turned down right away. The offering of my phone number was accompanied by a variation of a standard line I used at the time, "You're going to need this number one day. Maybe not tomorrow, or next week, but one day when he gets so comfortable that he really believes no other man wants you but him." I would always give a woman a husband or a boyfriend in my conversation, even though I knew many really had nobody.

I continued with my main theme, "Sweetheart, I'm what you might call a problem-free diversion. I'm not very aggressive and persistent, but I believe I have a lifestyle and a program that you can avail yourself of... on a limited basis. I love the city, I like going places, doing things — concerts, plays, and I'm really into blues and jazz. I'm political, an activist, and a black nationalist. I like to eat out in nice places, and I don't take myself too seriously. Keep this number for at least two weeks. Call one day to say hello. You know, you've made a new friend tonight, and things might never go beyond friendship, but you seem like the kind of woman who can have men friends."

Years later, Cyn said she had thought about giving a big, arms-stretching, wide-mouth, long yawn, right in the middle of my speech. I said that my recollection was of a woman awed and speechless. Anyway, I told her that night not to pass on my phone number to a lonely girlfriend. It was not just for anybody; she had been chosen.

"Now Cindy if you're absolutely positive you don't want to make the call... tear the number up, but please not in my face. At least, wait until I leave."

She just stood there looking pretty as a picture, a pleasant half-smile on her face, holding her daughter's hand. I had no idea she had such a quick wit, and that she was poised, like a snake, waiting to cut me down. I was all pumped up. I had walked up from the bar about four doors down, and a few drinks had me smoothly mouthing my lines, so I headed to the finale.

"Now, if you do decide to call, I'll expect the common courtesy I would extend to you if I called you. The act of simply asking in the beginning, 'Are you busy?', and of course if you said 'Yes,' I would simply say, 'I'll get back to you at a later time.' You see I'm extremely sensitive about interfering at the wrong time. This is a part of my being a problem-free diversion."

I just knew I was on a roll when she finally said, "And you're busy very often, right?"

I was about to say, "Well not really, because I'm very selective," but I couldn't get to anything before she said, "Probably busy calling your broker."

It stopped me cold. I was thinking, "What the hell is she talking about?" But before I could speak again, she said, "Or... are you broke, calling the loan company?"

I couldn't do anything but laugh and shake my head. Then I tried to come back, "Is that your way of asking me to pay for the chicken?" I accidentally had shown a little annoyance in my voice, so I quickly added, "So you're a comedian."

She said, "Aren't you?"

I had to use the little girl to get out of this, "Is Mommy mean to you like this sometimes?"

Then I had to make a quick switch in strategy. For some reason I knew instantly that I really wanted this woman, and it was light, begging time. "Look, you need to call my number more than I thought you did. Some guy has really got you bitter against all men, but I'm willing to forgive you anyway. Now, can I expect your call soon?"

She said, "I'll think about it."

"That's the best I can get?" I asked.

"I'll think about it seriously."

I leaned toward her ear and whispered, "You know I wouldn't really be heartbroken, but I'd be deeply disappointed if you didn't eventually call. Don't throw it away. Keep it for two weeks. If you lose it, I'm in the phone book. Ask Carol to get it, or you know where I work. Be good to yourself. Do yourself a favor, and make that call…you won't ever regret it."

I was always running down lines, even though I knew they were just dressing up a conversation. Most women, to a degree, have made up their minds in the beginning of a conversation as to whether they want to deal with you or not. In many hits, a man could be super-smooth, talk all day, and still get nowhere. I really figured that a line could blow your game more often than help it, but what the hell, I was at least entertaining myself.

When I was back on the barstool with the boys, I was thinking to myself, "Gamble, how did you let this younger, ex-student stop your well-used, smooth rap? She shoulda been awed by your experience, your superior street knowledge."

Anyway my mind was made up! "The woman needs me … and she's gonna get me."

She called two weeks later.

ColorStruck

primeval, aesthetical,
creative, discerning,
        Ms. Nature
is an artist, and she
has painted the Earth
with beautiful colors.

in pastels, in chroma
in spectrum, in tones
        and complexions;

so many pretty things
magnetically colorful,
like butterflies
        like wildflowers
like sunsets
        like gemstones
like autumn leaves
        like colored girls.

Being Alone

I find myself disconnected
every once in awhile and
these urges from somewhere
inside begin to disturb me
because what was full had
        become empty.

It was satisfaction and joy
that overflowed the spaces
        where they were,

        quickly
the spaces filled again
but with unfulfillment
uneasiness and melancholy.

I really need to be part of
        a twosome,
not just desirous of mating
        but desiring of a mate.

        It's more
than wanting, it's primal,
more than longing wistfully
it's original, fundamental
it's a hunger too essential
        to be ignored
just can't go on being alone.

Single Parents

Starting with my mother, I've been around intelligent, educated, progressive women all of my life. I can recognize one virtually at first sight because they emit this aura of irrepressibleness and inner-direction. They're just my type, and I mesh very well with them. I knew that Cynthia was my type when I first looked at her. She had that aura about her, and even more pleasing, it was all wrapped in a delicate-looking, pretty package.

Cynthia was twenty-six in 1975 when I met her. She was a newly divorced single parent with a son and a daughter. She was an independent woman. She was working at the telephone company, raising her kids, and going to college at the same time. She started out in college at Langston University, but she was finishing up work on her B.S. degree at Roosevelt University in Chicago. I worked for the Chicago Board of Education, and I had been divorced for a little over a year. I have a son, Oronde, but I really didn't become a single parent until he came to live with me the summer of 1987. That was the summer before he entered high school.

When I saw a woman that I knew I would like to get to know better, I was only disappointed if she was married. She had to be single, and that could mean single with or without children. So I was unfazed by knowing that Cyn had two kids, because I believed that if a man accepts the woman, he should accept her children. They are part of her.

They're the Earth Mother's primary responsibility. I didn't ever see myself in competition with a woman's children. I believed they should be first in her life, and she should work the man in her life around them. As the years went by in my relationship with Cyn, her daughter called her often when she was at my place. Sometimes Cyn would hang up the phone and say, "I got to go home."

Some of those times I was disappointed as hell at her leaving, but I would always say cheerfully, "All right, babe, I'll miss you."

Cyn worked for Illinois Bell (Ameritech) throughout the years we were together, and she was constantly striving to make a better life for herself and her kids. I was making more money than she was when I first met her, but she was moving up in the company, and she caught up with me fast. I would never concede that she ultimately outgrossed me. I would always say, "I'm off all summer, two weeks every Christmas, spring break for a week, an average of ten other holidays in the year, and I work a six-hour day."

It was all in jest, of course. We were not in competition about money or jobs because we knew we couldn't do each other's job. Besides from that, she really made out on my holidays. When I was off, that meant she could sleep later because I would drive her to work.

Cyn was always looking for a bigger and better apartment. I helped her move twice, and each place was bigger and better. She was adamant about having a nice place to live and for her kids, Jason and Crystal, to bring their friends over. She had great taste in furniture, and she reminded me of my mother by buying expensive things that lasted. Though she was always looking for a nice, safe place to live, she was even more aggressive about education. Cyn was always fighting to get her kids in the best schools.

In Chicago there's always an elementary school within walking distance of wherever you live, but she would by-pass that school to get her kids into a better one. Like a lot of other parents in Chicago who value a good education and safety, Cyn used every scheme she could to get her daughter into one of the top five public high schools. Her son was a top student who got into a magnet elementary school, and he attended the best college prep high school in the city, Saint Ignatius.

Cynthia's children were in no way a hindrance to our relationship; they were a joy to me in many ways. We liked each other, and I believe from my side it was because I'm from a big loving family that loved children. I had a son, many nieces and nephews, and there were a lot of kids by my first cousins, which were all a part of a big, loving, extended family. When we would go to my mama's house in Montgomery on many Thanksgivings, Cyn's daughter would fit right in. Her son opted to stay at home with his grandmother because they were very close. Some grandparents will practically take over the first grandchild as their own. Another reason I got along with her kids well was because I had learned not to play daddy with somebody else's kids. Children these days barely want to listen and obey their own parents, let alone some strange man. I just wanted to be their friend.

Cyn and I did take pot shots at each other's child-rearing methods. My boy was almost four when I met her. She went out with us sometimes when I picked him up on the weekend. She would complain that I allowed him to run wild in the stores. My thinking was, why not? He was a boy and athletic, so I turned him loose. One time, when he was around six, he was playing with her kids at her house, and he jumped up and down on her son's bed until he broke the slats. That gave her the perfect opportunity to say, "I told you he was wild." He got mad at her for trying to corral him sometimes. I used to tell her that she was too easy on her daughter.

Her daughter thought she should have everything her mama had and then some.

It was fun watching and critiquing each other's parenting tactics. We didn't attack each other's methods too harshly, but it did get a little testy every once in a while.

When her kids were young, she used to keep the Christmas toys she bought at my apartment, and we would take them over to her place about three in the morning. That was a lot of fun for me. As a divorced father, I didn't get a chance to wake up with my own son on Christmas morning and see his expression as he opened the toys. I didn't get a chance to see Cynthia's kids open the toys either, but at least I got to carry her around shopping. I would always buy my boy something extra for Christmas that I kept in my apartment. This was like having two Christmas mornings, and my son was anxious to come over and see what else he had. Later I celebrated Christmas and Kwanzaa at my apartment, so he got the opportunity to celebrate both holidays.

Cyn's mother lived with her, and this was much more than having a live-in babysitter. It was not only an advantage to her social life, but it eased the burden of being a working mother. In most jobs in private industry, workers have to stay until the job is finished, and this is especially so in management. This meant unexpected late evenings for Cyn. There were also times she had to go on training seminars for the weekend. Other times, she had to go to a training facility in the suburbs or out of town for a few days or a week.

I could see that the lot of a single, working mother was a difficult one. So many burdens that were meant for two to share were on her shoulders alone. Still, like some other male observers, I approached this fact in a very indifferent manner. I recalled a song by Tina Turner that said, "You got what you wanted, now you don't want what you got." At that time I agreed with a lot of the guys saying that many of these women should just crawl back to their husbands; it was too rough for them on their own. But when I stopped and analyzed the situation seriously, I became very sympathetic with the tough roles they were coping with. I wanted to be a joy to Cynthia; I wanted to help relieve some of the pressures on her. I absolutely didn't want to be another problem for her.

My family liked Cynthia from the first time I brought her home to Montgomery. They thought she was very personable and sweet for a Chicago girl. They grew to love her over the years, and my mama and daddy thought of her as another one of their daughters-in-law well before we were married. My brothers, in jest, tried to make me a married man because they were married but I always fought against assuming that title. Cyn was very close to my brother's wives, and as far as the family was concerned, she was my soulmate. And we would get married someday.

Today, I feel closer to Cynthia's children, Jason and Crystal, than I've ever been. They'll always be my stepson and stepdaughter, and I'll always look out for them as though they were my own.

Think About Me

She sent me a
Hallmark personal touch card,
it expressed exactly what she
wanted to say because it was
exactly what I wanted to hear.

She signed the love poem
"see you soon, love, Cynthia
P.S. — think about me."

The card was
loving enough but made more so
by her handwritten note which
stays in my head.

I'm still wondering about her
inner thoughts while penning
"think about me,"

was it just a passing thought?
a request? maybe a command?

it's enigmatic in my psyche
and important for me to know
because it defines me so well,
who I am, my daydreams.

Years ago
she scribbled "think about me."
and more than
ever I think somehow she knows,
it's all I ever do.

Serious Fun and Games

There were many available partners in the 1970s decade due to the surging divorce rate. A lot of men and women were reintroduced to the dating scene, and they just wanted to meet somebody nice to go out with. I was involved with several women that I dated more than once. Very few divorcees wanted to get married again right away, so some liaisons lasted only for a date or two. Others lasted for months and years, and some led to marriage.

During the sixties, women became more assertive; their assertiveness was at another level by the 1970s. A woman would quickly let a man know that she was an "independent woman." The expression showed how much women had been discriminated against. Guys didn't ever say, "I'm an independent man." It was an assumption made even when the guy was underemployed and still living at home with his mama. In the mid-1970s, women didn't just use the phrase "independent woman" as a cliche; it was a proclamation that they could take care of themselves, but it had much broader implications that a suitor was supposed to recognize.

When I started dating Cynthia, I was in the last stages of a relationship that had lasted over a year There was genuine affection between us, and we used the language of love. But neither of us felt that "this is it" and we could see our futures without each other. When liaisons like this were over, couples still could be mostly friends unless somebody really stepped on the other's ego.

I knew Cynthia was dating someone else, too, when we started seeing each other, because we couldn't always coordinate our dates. I had an encounter with the man she was dating without knowing who he was. He was a policeman, and he apparently had turned the corner when I was dropping her off in front of her apartment. After I pulled away, he stopped me a couple of blocks later for allegedly ignoring a stop sign. It was one of those "pull over and show your license" type of things. Cops can get a license plate check to find out your name and address, but I guess he just wanted to look me in the face. Cynthia told me a few days later who he was. She said she was livid when he revealed to her my name and where I lived. She was genuinely apologetic for the policeman's brazenness. I took it as a sign she was liking me more. It bothered me a little because I thought policemen were dangerous; many had the John Wayne complex. After Cyn revealed her relationship with him, I milked the incident for all I could get out of it.

"So...you're putting my life on the line, huh?" I even lied to her that he had thrown me against the car and frisked me illegally. "How could you deal with a cop like that?" I asked her. It was a diversion I needed at the time because I was really beginning to fall for Cynthia. But she kept reminding me that I wasn't serious about her; she claimed I was heavily involved with another woman. The other woman I was dating at the time lived three blocks from Cyn, and Cyn passed her apartment every day to catch the Illinois Central train to the Loop. She told me that she had seen my car parked in front of this apartment building too many times. It seemed as though every woman I met lived in the small South Shore area where I lived and socialized. Because Chicago is a big city I had stopped dating women who lived on the west side, or far away in general. But no matter how close Cyn and the other woman lived to each other, I was not about to drop one woman cold for another. I was a single man, just divorced. My policy was to add women, not to drop them. Although, if I had to move on, I thought it was best to gradually let a relationship wind down without anybody's feelings getting hurt. The "boys" always said to never quit a woman, but to let her quit you. That way it was easier to come back if you wanted to.

For a while I was dating Cyn and the other woman on a fifty/fifty basis (I'm going to call her "Ms. Goodum"). They had time to date others too. I suspected that they did, and it wasn't a big concern to me. To make things run smoother for myself, I saw one woman on Mondays, Wednesdays, and Fridays, and the other on Tuesdays, Thursdays, and Saturdays. I used to tell the Boys that I was like the Lord, and I rested on Sundays. Dating several women at the same time was a defense mechanism for me. Women could be as mercurial in relationships as men were, and if a man didn't want to get hurt, or get hurt as bad, he needed to have "a spare." I felt that a woman had the advantage in these types of situations, especially if she was a good-looking woman. Beautiful women are hit on all the time, and they could say yes to a date offer that had been coming in all along. For a guy in this situation at this time, if he didn't have somebody else, he couldn't get anybody, at least not right away. Comparatively speaking, it was drought time. Even the most undesirable women would turn you down.

Dating two women took a toll on me psychologically, financially, and physically. It soon occurred to me that this type of an arrangement didn't work out in my favor. Somehow in this situation, women always know about each other, and they seem to relish competition. They have all sorts of claiming rituals: leaving something personal in a man's apartment, marking his body with hickeys, and sometimes even confronting the other woman.

Basically, I was a guy waiting to naturally gravitate toward the woman I wanted the most. I would be correct in saying that I was really a one-woman man if I really loved the woman, the feelings were mutual, and the relationship was tight.

I knew I was getting close to Cynthia when she took me to meet her best girlfriend, Lynn. This is a man's first big test that comes before he can even dream about meeting her mama. Sometimes if these best girlfriends don't like you, you're out of the picture. I always felt that women give their girlfriends excellent advice concerning the men in their girlfriend's life, although for some reason they can't do nearly as well with the men in their own lives. Anyway, Cyn put the value of me meeting her best girlfriend and impressing her on the same level as having an audience with the Pope. It's mostly a casual affair with most men, and we feel that it's not what they think about us, but what we think about them. Still, I wanted to get a passing grade, even though I had just planned to be myself.

I met Cynthia in the fall of 1975, and her girlfriend came to visit her during the Christmas holidays of that year. I had gone to Montgomery to spend the holidays with my family, but had come back early to be with Cynthia. She introduced me to her girlfriend, Melba, from their college days at Langston University in Oklahoma. It wasn't a problem coming back to town early just to go out with Cyn. I simply didn't call the other woman I was dating until a few days later.

By this time I was falling fast, and Cyn and I went out several nights. She asked me about going out on New Year's Eve. Even though I wanted to be with Cyn, I wasn't dog enough to just break off my date with the other woman on a night as important as New Year's Eve. I was sort of stammering with a very apologetic type of an excuse to Cyn when she interrupted with, "Wait a minute. Are you saying you already have a date? That's cool with me. I know somebody else. I just thought you might have wanted to go out." I was both relieved and highly pissed off at the same time. You know, sort of jealously thinking to myself, "Who in the fuck does this woman think she's playing?" But I had the perfect solution. Cyn knew about the other woman, but the other woman didn't know about her. Cyn wanted to go out with me, and I wanted to go out with her. Here was a great situation for sisterhood to come into play. Cyn should have sympathized with my position and with the feelings of a sister. She should have given me the utmost respect for not just coldly breaking off my date, and file it in her memory bank as one of the perks she would receive once we were tight. Her next step should have been to wait at home alone on New Year's night with the hope that I would get rid of the other woman quickly. I would have made a maximum effort to do so. I would have secretly called her a couple of times and eventually gotten away, even though it would have been very early in the morning. Of course, I realize this scenario is much too fair for the average woman's nature. Anyway, in the scenario I envisioned, everybody would have been happy… especially me.

Melba was one of Cyn's super-smart and intensely spiritual girlfriends. She had a lot of them. I always enjoyed meeting and relating to so many sharp, intelligent women. Melba is a school psychologist. We stayed at her house when she was working in Atlanta, and she was driving a yellow BMW. When I was around Cyn's friend Lynn, a dentist, I thought she was always looking into my mouth. I thought Melba was always analyzing everything I said and analyzing everything Cyn told her about me. A guy can't help but feel a little strange, if not intimidated, when he is in the presence of two good-looking, intuitive women, especially if one is a psychologist. I know that Cynthia relied on Melba a lot for advice about child rearing and other problems in her life.

The time came when I simply wasn't enjoying the clandestine and deceptive nature of two half-way serious relationships, nor did I play them well. This game-playing is the essence of what it's all about to some guys. But I didn't pay much attention to strategy, details, and deceptive. I was the type of guy that would inadvertently tell on himself. To women, this was a crime within itself; an indictment of a man as an operator. Most women figure that a man will most definitely play around, but he should at least be slick enough to keep it out of their face. A while ago, one time after I had messed up overtly, a girlfriend told me, "Look, you don't know how to handle your business. You need to get your slow, country ass married, and stay home."

I think that's why a lot of the brothers go running to women of different nationalities. You got to have your shit together to master a true sister.

Occasionally, I would go for advice to that council of misinformation, "the boys." I didn't know a single man who didn't pose as an expert on how to handle women and how to handle multiple affairs. A man could pick up a few good points, but what worked for one guy did not necessarily work for another. Still, there was never any shortage of advice, solicited or not. Of course, if you really were in dire need for some good, sound advice; none was forthcoming. On the other hand, getting advice from one woman was getting it from five, going all the way back to their great grandmama.

I really didn't like being clandestine, sneaking around, going through all of the problems of keeping a relationship secret.

It's nothing like a beautiful, one-on-one love affair. I wanted to be happy and concentrate on making one woman happy. I couldn't fight off my growing feelings for Cynthia. I was definitely beginning to feel possessive.

I was hoping she would drop that clown she was dating. She was on the verge of picking up Mondays, Wednesdays, and Fridays if she moved quickly. But I decided I couldn't wait on her to write her own destiny; I would do it for her. I ended my other relationship with an Academy Awards performance. My show was probably not necessary because she had things going for herself, but she deserved to go out in style. My theme was, "I had given her my best shot." Still it was clear to me I could no longer make her happy. I understood why she was leaving me, and as heartbreaking as it was, I would somehow persevere. I figured that she already had another man in her life when she accepted my lie so fast.

About six weeks passed, and things were going great for me because I could give Cyn all of my time. For my old flame, apparently, her new thing didn't pan out as well as she thought it would. When she called me to possibly spend a night together, it blew my ego sky high. I was thinking, "Woman, I could have told you it takes a helluva man to follow me!"

My situation wasn't the same as before, because at that time I was really into Cynthia. Still, I had doubts. I wasn't certain whether Cyn had cut all of her ties with other men, and whether she was absolutely ready for an exclusive relationship. I may have been just playing mind games with myself, because my ego kept telling me to go ahead and give this old flame a few hours, "Gamble, go ahead and let her see what she's been missing."

I knew it was the wrong move the minute she sat in my car. She was looking really good, but all of the sparks between us were in the past, and I knew she felt the same way. Whenever Cyn opened my car door and slithered in beside me, I was always slammed with her sensuality and femininity. It was as if just seconds before, she had put on her face perfectly, and she had read me perfectly. Her smile and stare arrogantly said to me, "All right boy, I know you want me, so it's OK to show more enthusiasm and aggressiveness." And I did, but whenever she first got into my car I was immobile, infatuated, and unable to take the car out of park until she came closer and placed her tongue in my mouth.

I really didn't see myself as any big prize, although I knew I was nowhere near the worst dude out there. I didn't trip off the episode because I realized that women will compromise themselves to win, but that's less about the man and more about competition between women.

As for the rendezvous, if it was anything it was sad, and

we didn't need to say hardly anything about our relationship being permanently over. We had once been to a beautiful tropical island together. Now the cheap motel said it all. But that's life... sometimes you leave somebody, and sometimes somebody leaves you. What made it really bad was that I missed my chance to use the line I always wanted to use at the end of a relationship. I'm a romantic and a movie buff. I always liked the ending scene from "Casablanca." I wanted to paraphrase Humphrey Bogart's parting line about Paris and say, "Baby, I know we can never be together again as lovers, but we'll always have the ghetto."

I was happy the relationship ended with less pain than any other I've been in. It's not too often that two people want to move on basically around the same time. I think it had a lot to do with there being so many divorcees; only a few wanted to get serious. I know I didn't want to get serious, but I didn't want to live in the fast lane either. A guy can get a lot of props for being fast, but being fast is really no great feat. It's a very easy game to play if you want to play games. All you had to do was not be concerned about somebody else's feelings, and the other things just followed. I ran with a lot of fast guys; I knew how the game was played, and like any other thing in life, you can learn how to do it well even if it's not your second nature.

I had a philosophy and game plan for me to be happy. I wasn't interested in getting married or even staying with a woman who wanted to get married. I appreciated being a bachelor more than bachelors who had never been married. This doesn't mean that I was totally hardened against the institution of marriage, because I wasn't. I think it's a mistake to go into a relationship for the purpose of getting married. I was looking for a good, stable relationship, which might or might not turn into marriage. Marriage is a very serious business. To me, it wasn't about security or status. Even though they're not mentioned that much in reference to men, they are the reasons a lot of guys get married. After all, there are more African-American women with middle-class credentials than there are African-American males. I wanted to make sure my marriage lasted forever this time. I wanted it to be based mainly on deep, undying love for a woman I couldn't see myself living without. I couldn't possibly determine this in a short period of time. I believe in lust at first sight, but not love at first sight. Meanwhile, I wasn't interested in running the streets with a string of simultaneous surface relationships either. I just wasn't going to allow an orgasm to hold me in involuntary servitude.

I wanted to find a woman I could mesh with as the first step toward love. Logic says the best type of relationship is one that eliminates the negatives of the married life and the single life. A blend of the best qualities of each would be ideal, and that was the main goal of my game plan.

If this isn't a morally indefensible position, I would say that the mid-seventies was a great time to be divorced. It was much better for men who were not control freaks. As the change in relations between men and women picked up speed, a lot of guys didn't accept it, or they just couldn't recognize the change. On the other hand, I thought I was a careful observer of trends, and the trends of the mid-seventies told me that we were in a new era in relationships with women. A lot of independent women said they didn't want to get married. I took them at their word, but I half-way believed that it was a reaction to the shortage of available males or their own high standards. Either way, many women didn't get married. Still, for a man to believe that all women want to get married isn't a totally foolish assumption. A totally foolish assumption is to believe that all women want to get married to him. So my mind was at ease, because I wasn't stuck on myself enough to believe that every woman I dated wanted to marry me.

The traditional two-parent family was in transition, and the female-headed family was in ascendancy. From a hierarchical standpoint, I saw this as a woman's children being her first consideration, she was second, and the man in her life was third. I could definitely live with this set-up. So Cindy seemed like a good relationship for me. She was an independent woman who didn't even joke about getting married. A woman who had her priorities straight because I was third. She didn't have time for me everyday, and she couldn't stay overnight most of the times. I wouldn't have respect for a woman who placed a man, myself included, over the interest of her children. I never ran into this type of woman. All of the women I dated with children were good mothers first. They knew the right things to do and what not to do in front of their children. This is one of the main problems of divorced women with children. I had seen Cynthia with her daughter on the second time that we met, but it was months before she invited me to her apartment to officially meet her mother, son, and daughter.

Sometimes what starts out as just fun and games can turn serious without warning. I knew I wanted somebody, and I was looking for somebody. Maybe not looking for a wife, but a soulmate. I had found her, and I knew it.

PBT

It
was in autumn, not spring
she was fresh on the scene
I threw my hat in the ring
I needed another plaything.

Life's
full of things unforeseen
she quickly broke down my
scheme,
I blinked and she's first
string,
paused and she was my
queen.

It
was a whole 'nother thing
I'm jealous and starting to
cling,
buying gold hoop earrings

she's got me taking ginseng.

I wanna sing, wanna scream
I wanna give her a diamond
ring,
want everything she brings

she's one pretty-black-thing.

The Source of the Light

The light
is sentimental and stirring
the light is close, caressing,
I'm basking in a glow
of warmth and loving feelings
powerless to resist.

I have to
find the source of the light
for it is incandescent soft
and it's natural as the dawn,

but I know it's not the sun.

The light
is intense, but not flaming,
it's an even tepid fervor,
I know it's not from a fire,

flickering intermittently
it's a wondrous illumination,

like a thousand fireflies

on a dark steamy summer night
and I'm sure it's not the
Tiffany lamp on my nightstand
left turned on during bedtime.

The light
shines, penetrates through me
and I'm bashful, but desiring,

and
the light reads all that I am
but it's not radiation though
it is naturally radiant.

One dark transcendental night
it just all came to me calmly,

the source of the light

it's that jubilant sparkle
in her eyes when she smiles,

that
sunshiny dancing in her eyes
when she's laughing, sassing.

It's that
candle from her look of love

and the
light is innocently seducing
for she is unassumingly sexy
just being her natural self.

To Have Somebody

Looking for love is a fascinating game. It's an exciting time, unless it becomes neverending. Then it's like playing your favorite sport over and over, but losing all the time. Winning is ending up having somebody. I really enjoyed those days when I was in pursuit of Cynthia, and I expected it to end exactly the way it ended.

I've heard a good number of people say that they don't need another to be complete. I can't even begin to understand what they mean, unless they're saying that they don't need anybody at any cost. Or that a person should not accept anybody, just to have somebody. I need somebody. I guess I'm a lot like the first man, Adam. I can live in paradise, but without a woman to love and to love me, I would be incomplete and lonely.

Although it wasn't love at first sight for Cyn and me our "like affair" turned quickly into a love affair. Both of us were romantic activists. We liked doing all of those ritualistic things normally associated with courtship. Rituals like going places, doing things together, impressing one another, being impressed, and giving and taking. I wanted it to go even farther because I enjoy the trappings of being deeply in love. I was hoping things would progress to the point when I knew who I was going to be with on Christmas Eve and who was going to take me out for my birthday dinner.

I wanted to reminisce about her in my daydreams, and it came to pass. When I wasn't with her, those lapses in my attention span were watching her painting on lipstick and combing her hair in the mirror of my mind. At first I thought I was the hunter, but she always made me feel like I was the prey. It must have been that both of us were hunters, and both of us were prey. And that accounted for how quickly we reached the point where we could say that we had somebody.

Nevertheless, maybe it was just me and maybe not. It could just be the nature of the relationship, but I clearly recall a feeling I had at the time. The external forces that were in our way, we had gone through, stepped over, and finally vanquished. And I really felt that we were one. Still, I was being stalked by uncertainty or the feeling of "now what?"

I wasn't sure how things would turn out even though I believed we could go beyond the initial good feelings of any new relationship. I had fallen in love. I was on a high, riding the tidal wave, but for how long? It was that turning point, a time when it seemed that all that was standing before me were a lot of questions. Is the game over, or has it just begun? Is the pursuit the most exciting and happiest part of a union? Will romance now take a beating? What does she really want of me, and what can I give?

I wanted some fast and definitive answers. At least that's what I kept telling myself. I knew the main answer; I just didn't want to deal with it. I was afraid of commitment. Women that say a lot of men are afraid of commitment are right. Of course I was scared. It was a lot like wanting to be "saved," but not wanting to totally live the religious life, or being afraid that I couldn't totally live that life.

It's really hard to let go of that great male illusion of being totally free. Plus, I had placed my heart in this woman's hand, and I had just known her for a year. I didn't like that feeling of vulnerability. And I figured Cyn had her doubts too. But even though I was afraid of commitment, it wasn't going to stop me from being committed. A state of fear is a part of love.

I was sitting at a bar having a drink when it hit me to turn off all of those unnecessary questions about longevity and the future because it's natural and very "male" to just enjoy things while they last. Excessive questions and fears seemed to me to be so female.

After a few Jack Daniel's, my cultural upbringing, chauvinism, and the N-word in me surfaced, washing away my doubts and fears. I sat there thinking a lot about myself. The kind of a man I was, my program, the type of lover I was, and I said to myself, "Leave ME? Shiiit! ...I'm the best thing that ever happened to the woman! Let the good times roll!"

I was confident that if Cyn really got to know me well, she would want to keep me for a while and probably even longer. I have this great capacity for love. I offered my love to Cindy, and she was smart enough to take it. It was the beginning of loving times for us, those days which I now call technicolor days. Just as I had planned it, we had managed to manipulate the best of the institution of marriage and the single life. This meant having a long love affair with a high level of romanticism. That wasn't a breeze; it needed fine tuning constantly. But you understand... it was a labor of love.

I know it wasn't just our relationship that took work because many people believe that living together sometimes destroys love and romance. Couples don't have to live in a cave together for protection anymore. Roles and rules born out of necessity have changed. There's no set family pattern as there were in the days when the man went out to hunt, and the woman stayed to watch the children and cook the meals. A lot of lovers believe it's not living together that's so hard on romance and love, it's saying "I do." But it's obvious that there are many, many, happily married couples, and they still have a lot of romance in their relationship. So

I guess each relationship should be tailor-made around some agreed-upon rationale by the couple. Cyn and I were in agreement on the type of relationship we had, and for 17 years we didn't say "I do" or live together. I firmly believe that for us, these two decisions were the foundation for the high level of romanticism and happiness we shared.

We had a great situation for us. She had her own place, I had mine. This worked out to both of our advantages. We always lived less than ten minutes away from each other by car, so picking her up and dropping her off was fast and easy. If there was an emergency at her apartment while we were at my apartment, I could have her home in no time.

The early stage of our relationship, of dating each other exclusively, was like any other hot and heavy relationship. It's that stage when a man seldom sees his girlfriend without her face on. We frequented movies, plays, concerts, lounges, and went out to dinner a lot. She seldom talked about her family situations. We grew close fast because she was sweet and funny; I was actually fighting myself from asking for more of her time. My type of romantic love is strongly blended with the altruistic Christian chivalry type of love. I make myself happy by being of service and making the woman in my life happy. This called for me to fight against my inherent selfishness and total independent spirit. I'm a willing compromiser up to a point, and somehow Cyn was intuitively in tune to that point. Some things that she liked to do she would just drop because she knew I didn't want to do them. Other things she pushed, whether I wanted to do them or not. And she was an expert at using the art of dropping the old guilt trip on a man.

A bachelor with his own place is an ideal situation for a female single parent. It's a love nest, a get-away spot, a bastion of privacy. And in talking about privacy, there is a narrow view and there's a broad view. In a boyfriend's home a woman didn't have to put her hands in dishwater, vacuum, or referee children's disputes. There was food, drinks, soft music, adult conversation, or golden silence. When Cyn got a chance to stay at my place overnight, she could dress for work, or I could quickly have her home in time to shower and dress for work. I believe the broad view of privacy for a female single parent is to not to have her life totally dominated and completely immersed in the child rearing culture. The adult culture was king at my place. It was a place where our friends could meet and socialize. For Cynthia, it was a home away from home, and for us, it was our home.

In our separate residences, the stress and negatives of living together were eliminated, and a lot of mundane things were altered into something pleasant. When regulated, even just sleeping together becomes something desired, missed, and longed for. The "space" that everybody talks about needing every once in a while can also be regulated. We were masters at giving each other needed space. Many people didn't know that we were so close because we were not up under each other all of the time. Having a great sense of humor helped our relationship a great deal. We were able to say to each other what some might consider too sensitive to talk about. We regulated certain routines without hurting any feelings. Mostly, in a hot and heavy love affair, lovers naturally want to be together a great amount of time. But there are also times when you want to just check in over the telephone and see each other the next day or a few days later. Cyn had an excellent excuse for needing space time because she lived with her family, had to share her time, and she had more responsibilities. When I needed space, I had to make sure not to send the wrong signals. A lot of women believe that time away from them is time with another woman. Although, just as absence makes sleeping together a treat, sleeping together all the time makes sleeping alone a treat. As a bachelor, I had this comfort zone of living alone and being alone without being lonely. I liked getting back to my zone every once in a while, no matter how much I loved a woman. I believe many women feel this way too, but it's a situation that is so misunderstood in relationships, because it could be a signal that you're just getting bored with each other.

We instituted policies. The phrase "I'm going to call it a night" meant I'm going to stay home, and I'll call you tomorrow. When one of us really needed to be with the other on a particular day or night, the expression was, "You got to pay some dues." The days in between the times we didn't see each other served to increase that longing feeling. Those days kept our relationship fresh. Most of the time we couldn't go more than two days without touching each other. If it was a Monday and she could not stay overnight until the weekend, we had to see each other if only for a short while. I would drive to her apartment building and wait for the chartered bus she rode to and from work. Many times she called and asked me to meet the bus or to drive to the Loop so we could ride back to the South Shore together.

I think the biggest advantage in her having her own place and me having mine were those times when there were serious debates. The only sure way to avoid debates or arguments in a relationship is for one of the partners to have absolutely no thoughts or opinions of their own. We were both independent thinkers; this meant some bitter debates sometimes. I prefer to use the term debates over arguments because we established boundaries. We were easy-going and civilized, so we never resorted to loud, profane, name-calling viciousness. We were divorcees and didn't believe in arguing about third parties; that was a separation issue. In principle, we agreed that if either one of us wanted somebody else or felt cramped, we would just let the other one know. This, of course, works better in theory than in practice, so I was happy we were never put to the test.

As we moved past our second year together, having our separate residences was really working to our advantage. I'm known to get on a woman's nerves sometimes. Cyn wasn't about to just take it. She would quickly say, "Take me home," or she would just put on her coat and leave. Twice, she even asked me to pull the car over, and she took the CTA bus home. (That was an argument, not a debate!) I really hated that, and she knew how it got on my nerves. I convinced her that when we argued, to just let me take her home safely, and we could take it from that point. She finally agreed.

I've said that our relationship had a high level of romance, and that it was achieved through constant fine tuning.

Sometimes it was from my side, and other times from hers. One Friday evening after I picked up Cyn and brought her to my place, I noticed how bone-tired she looked. After she had taken off her coat I asked, "What do you want to eat? I wanna get it before we get comfortable. You really look tired, babe. Come over here, sit down, and tell Daddy all about it."

She came over, sat beside me, gave me a lazy kiss, and put her head on my chest. She was talking slowly, "Bob I'm tired. I want to change places with you."

"Cyn, you're taking that penis envy thing too far; you wanna be a man now."

"Don't be silly. I want the privileges and advantages of a man."

"So you wanna be a white man. You don't mean a man like me, a black man catching hell in America."

"That's better than a black woman catching double-hell because she's a woman."

"Cyn, I know you're not going to fuck up this evening talking feminist shit. Sure you're tired. Y'all wouldn't listen. We tried to tell you feminists that the workplace was a bitch. It's just like that song said… you got what you wanted, now you don't want what you got."

She asked me to move down on the sofa, so she could stretch out and place her head in my lap. Looking up at me she said, "If we changed places, you wouldn't last two months. Like…really, Bob, what do you do?"

"What do I do? I work like you do."

"What do you do after work? I'm a divorced woman and you're a divorced man. You have a son, like I have my children, but where is your son tonight? Did you help him with his homework? Did you have to take him to the doctor this week? Did you have to make dinner like I did for my kids and mother? My mother's almost 70, and I can't even trust her to cook anymore because she forgets to turn off the pots." And she went on and on talking about all of the things a single-parent, working-mother has to deal with.

"OK Cyn, I understand, but what in the hell brought this on?"

"You did."

"What!"

"Not today. The other day when I asked you to pick me up from work."

"And I did pick you up."

"But you didn't like it, and you were quiet all the way back because you were missing some game."

"I was listening to the game on the radio."

"Bob, you gave me a dry kiss when I got in the car, and you hardly said anything else. I asked you to come down because I wanted to be with you. I wanted us to have a pleasant ride home. How many bosses do you have on your job that you have to impress? I needed my man to be happy to see me and happy to be with me."

I was thinking to myself, "Another masterful Cyn guilt trip, but two can play this game."

"Cyn that's unfair. I take you every place you need to go and every place you want to go. Some discount shoe store way out in the suburbs. I even give up sleeping late on my holidays, so you can sleep late, and then I drive you to work."

"Bob, I know you're a good man. I can depend on you, and you do a lot of things for me ... but..."

I was quick, "But what!"

"I would like for you to be more pleasant."

"Cyn you can't be serious. You know I'm not moody, and nobody's ever accused me of being so. I'm a fun guy."

"I like you to be more pleasant when you're doing things for me that you may not like or want to do at the time."

I had to laugh. I was scratching my head looking up, "Let me see... The Lord loves a cheerful giver, and Cyn loves a cheerful dues payer."

"Bobby, I do a lot of things for you I'm not thrilled about doing, but I always try to be pleasant about them. Look, you have two simple choices. You can say yes or no. If you say yes, then you should at least try to be pleasant."

"You have two simple choices, too. You can do it yourself, or ask me to do it. If you decide to ask me, you should accept that I can't possibly be chipper about it all the time."

I made a quick point about choices I had made which I thought evened us up, but I immediately felt that I was being too callous. She didn't drive, so she needed me. Everything she could do for me, she did. She would always greet me smiling, or she had the look of love in her eyes. But I was just as upbeat as she was, if not more so, and I say this because I had much fewer responsibilities and other reasons to be in a down-mood swing. However, there were two areas which could usher in my silent treatment. That was when I had to miss part of a game I really wanted to see, and when I missed my favorite television program. This was in the late seventies before a VCR solved that predicament. I was also impatient when Cyn was late. I didn't fuss; I was just quiet. Cyn was catty as hell about it sometimes, asking me, "Are you on your period tonight?"

I made a quick reversal that night. I remember the night

well because of how tired she looked, how sincere she sounded, and the realization it brought concerning the difficulties she faced as a single-parent and a working mother. She wasn't a super woman as Karyn White says in her song, "Super Woman." Cyn was as strong as she had to be, but she wasn't as strong as she appeared to be. There was delicacy and vulnerability underneath her shield of the strong, independent woman. She told me her life was much tougher than mine, and she was absolutely right. I knew it was, but she went into more detail than she had before.

Cyn wasn't asking much of me, just for me to be a little more understanding. To be more patient and pleasant when paying relationship dues. The night touched me deeply. Although I was never perfect, from then on it was always on my mind to try harder. To take off that negative, emotional surtax I placed on some of the things I would do for her. I knew I was sweet to her, but I could be even sweeter, and I was. Throughout the years, she would always ask me why was I so good to her.

Cyn's head was still resting in my lap, and after a quick kiss on the mouth I said, "All right babe, I'll be more pleasant, but it's going to cost you to do something very special for me."

She let out a long sigh. "What now Bobby?"

"You're going to have to learn how to make banana pudding, and it has to be this weekend. In fact, I want some tomorrow when I pick you up, or if I pick you up. You know how I love banana pudding."

She reluctantly agreed, "OK, I'll try."

I had to get us something to eat, and on Friday nights in Chicago, it's a southside ritual to eat some delicious barbeque ribs. Chicago has the best ribs in the country. I was going to go get us some, but before I would leave, I decided I wanted to hear something. I was close enough for her to look into my eyes as if something were in one of them, and I needed her to gingerly blow it out, so in a serious manner, I asked, "Cyn before I leave, tell me what do you see in my eyes?"

"Buck shots! Perversion!"

"OK, you've gotten in your comedic line. Now...what do you see in my eyes?"

"Need."

"All right, I'll go along with that, but look deeper."

"Possessiveness, jealousy."

"Jealousy? Should I be? Woman, what do you see?"

"Bobby, I hope this is not your impression of a dreamy-eyed passionate look."

I was silent. So conjuring up a smile she said, "Infatuation."

"Look deeper."

Slowly and seriously, she said, "OK, baby...You really, really love me."

I didn't say anything else. I got up, headed for the door, then turned and gave her one of those winks she always gives me, and said, "You're damn right I do."

I couldn't knock Cyn about that night, because I expected mostly pleasantness out of her too.

I really preferred to use our separate residences in times of heavy disputes. Sometimes these were about nothing important, just the stress that comes with a relationship. Being a bachelor, I absolutely didn't want a woman in my apartment with her jaws tight, especially in my bed overnight. Women don't like you to touch them when they're mad, and most guys cool off after a couple of hours. Men want to get sweet again, but women don't cool off so fast. They stay mad sometimes for days. When Cyn was mad, she knew how to scrunch to the far side of the bed and fall into a deep sleep on the very edge of the bed. The only thing that would wake her was my moving just an inch toward her, so I had to really suffer because now more than ever I wanted to snuggle and touch.

I was unusually sleepy the next morning, and she was rested, refreshed, and still pissed off about something I could hardly remember. I just don't know how she could be mad as hell and still sleep peacefully. Anyway, I instituted this policy based on the fact that only married men have to take this quiet, jaws-tight, distant, evil woman in your bed bit.

I told Cyn, "If you can't be sweet and cuddly, I'll take you home until you can. This is a bachelor's lair, be sweet or be gone."

She answered, "I'll let you know if I want to ever see you again. Take me home."

"Sure babe, anytime you want, or even dream that you want."

Damn! I was talking big, but I missed just touching her that night. I knew I was going to catch hell, still I was determined not to be the one to call first. "Monday Night Football" got me through the first night. She was strongly on my mind all day Tuesday at work, but I still simply refused to call first. Wednesday, my mind began to rationalize on its own: "Gamble, this is stupid. You know you wanna call, so go ahead." I picked up the phone several times, then slammed it down, and went on to bed frustrated. Thursday, during my lunch period at work, my mind teamed up with my horniness, and together they won the rationalization game. I wanted to be with my baby. I missed her too much to continue this high school game. When I first called, she was out to lunch, so I left a message with the exact time that I was calling back.

When I got her on the line my conversation was aimed to convince her that I was only calling first to do her a favor,"OK Cyn, I decided you've suffered long enough. I'm taking you off punishment. I'm sorry I didn't return all of your calls or respond to your telegram, but I was busy. To make up for that I'm allowing you to forego your apology. You know how I hate to hear a woman begging."

She stopped me abruptly with, "Shut up fool! Be down in front of the building after work."

"All right sweet girl, I missed you baby."

"I missed you too, old man. You've been good?"

"Would I give away what belongs to you?"

"You're over the hill, but you probably tried. When are you going to get an answering machine? You're scared I'm going to listen to the tape?"

"You would do something like that."

"Look Bobby, I want some Chinese food tonight."

"Anything for you, sweet baby."

"And we'll have to stop by Walgreens and get some napkins."

"What! I know you're talking about dinner napkins."

"You know what type of napkins I'm talking about."

"Hell naw... You've got to be joking."

"Well, you should have called yesterday."

"Looks like I might have to see you in about five days."

"Bobby that's a cruel thing to say."

"I know. I'm sorry babe. I was just joking."

"You always go too far."

"OK sweet I'm really sorry, and I won't ask you if you were joking. I'll meet you about five. I love you sweetheart."

I don't know why women pick the wrong time to lose their sense of humor, but this called for something extra to get her back into a loving mood. So I stopped by Carson's while I was in the Loop, got some cologne, and looked for those guys in the street selling single red roses. Meanwhile, my mind was racing like hell trying to count back and pinpoint her cycle to see whether she was playing or not. All in all, it turned out to be another splendid week, and it was never a dull week... I had somebody!

Reflections on Having Somebody

When you have breezed through what
others consider a very hard day,
    you have somebody!

You're inwardly happy, though few
things presently are going your way,
    you have somebody!

Passing thru the women's store
    Carson Pirie Scott
surrounded by the various scents of
    perfumes and colognes
in dazzling hexagons, octagons, and
    cube-shaped bottles
gold earrings, silver bracelets, and
other prim, pretty, delicate things
    I can't help but think of her.

I was there shopping for myself but
it feels much better looking for,
finding, buying her a surprise gift
    I have somebody!

    I really didn't
want to go, but it made her happy,
    I have somebody!

Playoff game is close at the half
she's not expecting me today, but
I can't enjoy the game because it's
getting dark, she might have to wait
in the cold, I leave to pick her up,
    I have somebody!
(Of course, it's not a Bull's game.)

You walk into a room or
you're just strolling thru the mall
the beautiful people are everywhere
occasionally a
good-looking face will turn your way
friendly eyes ask are you available?

You glance back without thinking,
a mutual attraction, maybe? but you
keep moving, don't return the stare,
you have somebody!

Weekend finally arrives and you have
nothing specifically planned but you
are still expecting a good time,
you have somebody!

Xmas, Easter, Thanksgiving, birthdays
happy times are rolling around,
besides from family you want somebody
special to be with you, at your side,

start the hustle and bustle of planning,
pick up the turkey, get the Xmas gifts,
buy the Easter lilies and the valentine,
you have somebody!

I'm down to the very last slice of
this delicious sweet potato pie,
my mama made it for me Thanksgiving,
my mouth's watering, the craving is
just unbearable,
nobody should expect to get any of
your last piece, but I share it with her,
I have somebody!

I'm pissed off, she actually changed
        a hair style I really loved,
in just a week, I loved the new style
        much more than the other,
I had somebody, or did she have me?

When a stare can make a man shut up,
or behave, it's more about being in
love than weakness. He has somebody!

Loving, hot passion is overcoming me,
want to release, want to explode,
but I hang in there and wait on her,
        I have somebody!

        I insisted that
she learn how to make banana pudding
and I added, "Just like my mama's."
        I was being unfair,
she eventually did much better after
the first try when I ended up drinking
        the banana pudding;

        she couldn't explain that and I
was forbidden to ever mention it again,
I should have known that no girlfriend
soulmate, or even a wife can ever cook
        as good as a man's mama,

but everything turned out fine,
she came up with several spectacular
desserts that neither I, nor my mama
had ever heard of, but I would beg
        her to make them.
Bless her soul… I had somebody!

I Love You… I Love You, Too

I really love reminiscing and this is a week I can't forget. I hear some people say that it was love at first sight, and I think, "that really must be something." I wonder whether they're telling the truth, or just mistaking what that initial attraction actually was.

I think we all love at first sight, babies, material things, and beautiful things that make up the Earth and the sky. For me, I could be infatuated, or smitten at first sight, but real love is much more complicated.

For love, I would need time. There would have to be shared experiences, not just daydreaming. When she was not around, I would have to feel, taste, swallow her, and she would be floating through my veins. It would have to get to that point where I would claim I possessed her, but in reality, I knew she would possess me. If it was true love, she could change my life. And of course, there's a down side; unfortunately, with me being unable to prevent it, she would be able to break my heart.

But I don't focus too much on the negatives. Whatever it was that made me feel love was stalking Cynthia and myself, I turned to greet it. It was what I was looking for, and I'm not one to keep happiness waiting.

Still, in the relationship game, it's not easy for a man to know when it's really love, we're wrapped up in feelings of sexuality and possessiveness. These emotions are a part of love when it's real love, but they can stand alone, falling somewhere short of real love.

After months of dating and intimacy, I felt deeper feelings, but those feelings didn't crystallize into a moment when I just said to myself, "I love her." Maybe that's why I remember the events that led to me realizing that it was real love so well.

I was enjoying the moment. I was basking in that great feeling of not being totally committed to anything but my own happiness, and that's not a callous statement. When I first saw Cyn and sized her up, I didn't say to myself, "I want to make her happy." I wanted to make myself happy.

I know what love is. I had been married before and felt love on other occasions. It wasn't a case of me knowing that I loved her, but playing the relationship game of not wanting to say it first. For months, we had used every term of endearment one can use, short of out and out saying, "I love you."

I have this picture book of Cyn, and the first picture in it is the first picture she gave me. The story behind the picture is our first confession of love.

I was just moving along in our relationship, haphazardly as is my nature. I used to take a lot of pictures. Whatever woman was coming over to my apartment, I would place her picture on my dresser. You know give the lady a little personal touch.

I was expecting Cyn over. I had put her picture up, but for some unknown reason, I left the other woman's picture face down on the dresser.

When Cyn picked it up and looked at it, I quickly grabbed it from her hand.

"Sorry babe, I was just getting rid of this."

I felt I had to be dramatic, so I took the picture out and tore it into bits right in front of her. Then I said,

"I hope this doesn't seem cruel, but when it's over, it's

over." Of course, I had another copy.

Cyn was completely unimpressed and unamused. She looked at me intently,

"You have a decision to make."

"I've made my decision; this was just something I forgot to do."

Of course, when caught, a man should always attack,

"Since I've never been in your bedroom, I don't know whether you've made a decision, or not, but I'll take your word for it, if you say so."

Cyn could easily access that "feline aloofness" of a woman who has been told all of her life she was a pretty woman, and believed it. So she acted in a manner recognizing femininity as power. She knew she was a flower, I had tasted her nectar, and I wanted more. It was time to put me on punishment.

Everything about her that evening was perfect. She had changed from work clothes into a soft dress. Her face was perfect, and her hair was perfect. She didn't believe in splashing cologne on so heavily that it dominated the air. It was worn very lightly; I had to be very close to get a whiff of it. She was extra stunning that day, and it made my situation worse, because I knew I had fucked up and she was going to go home.

She said, "You need a few days to make up your mind about our relationship, if there's to be a relationship. I want you to take me home, but I don't want to talk about it in the car. Don't call me; you'll only make it worse. I'll call you when I figure the time is right."

In the car, I decided not to say anything, because I wasn't about to beg to a woman. In fact I was feeling downright arrogant. I always figured that getting another woman was never any problem for me. When I was feeling this way, I had this little game I used to play with myself to further pump myself up.

I would add an R to my last name and say to my self, "Don't sweat it brother. She must not know that you're Bob Gambler, the woman handler."

I said nothing, as Cyn had asked me to, and dropped her off. I was sort of pissed and for some reason I decided to call the woman in the picture I had torn up. I hadn't talked to her for a while, so when she picked up the phone, I decided to ask right off, was she busy? The bitch coldly said, "Yes."

Obviously, I have to put this day down on my top ten list of fucked-up days.

Fortunately for me, in those days I was still on the bar-hopping circuit. A bar is a good place to do some thinking or be distracted. Besides, I was trying to figure out what was wrong with Cyn. It wasn't like she had come across me with a woman in my bedroom. It was just a picture of another woman, and the picture was face down. If she hadn't turned it over, I certainly wouldn't have done so.

I hit the joints, mainly to get myself in a better mood. It was somewhat distracting, but I couldn't get her out of my head, especially the way she looked that Friday evening. And echoing in my ear was the sound of her voice: her laughter, whisperings, sighs, and moans.

That Wednesday I received a letter from her. Normally that's something pleasant, but as I was walking up to my apartment to open it, I was cursing to myself.

"Fuck it she ain't got the nerves enough to call, or come and say it to my face."

When I opened the letter, it was two blank sheets of paper wrapped around a beautiful picture of herself. Most people take a quick look at a picture and quickly turn it over to see if there's an inscription on the back. I did the same.

Today, it's the first picture in my picture book of Cyn. On the back it says, "Don't hide this one," and was signed

"Cynthia, I Love You."

I consider myself a poet, but I can't fully describe the feelings that came over me at that moment.

When I look up love in the dictionary, it doesn't mention the word joy, and I know that love can be a brooding feeling that's sometimes laced with pain. But as I read, "I love you" in her soft, feminine penmanship, it brought on that airy feeling of love. I was swept by a wind gust of joy. And it didn't pass quickly over me; I sat down because the joyous feeling lingered and lingered like an afterglow.

It was all so stunning. In less than a week, I had gone from one of my worst days to one of my happiest. I fixed myself a drink, put on some love songs, and relaxed on the sofa just basking in the joy. I got off work two hours earlier than Cyn, so I figured I had over three hours to come up with a nice response.

I wasn't the type of guy to just throw around the expression of "I love you" because it's something women wanted to hear. Also, in the middle seventies, many independent women would greet a guy's heartfelt expression of love with, "Wait a minute. I think we might be moving too fast." Then a guy would feel like a damn fool.

I spent the next few hours soaked with joy and thinking about how I was going to orchestrate what I had to say. Although I didn't play the player's role well, I was very good at being a man in love.

I absolutely was not going to use "too" as in "I love you too." And it was absolutely not to be said during pillow talk. I really wanted her to know that she may have said those words first, but I had been feeling them for some time.

I gave her a while to get settled down from work before I called. I had rehearsed what I planned to say, but it didn't come out exactly the way I wanted it to. But I was at least upbeat, short, to the point, and as slow and deliberate as I had planned.

"Hi! I got your letter, so I guess it's OK for me to call. I really would prefer to say what I have to say in person." She quickly interrupted with,

"It will have to be on the weekend. I'm tired."

Everything I had rehearsed was put on hold, so I had to say something impromptu,

"OK, I'll wait because I really would not like to say what I have to say on the phone. But that is two days off so for now, I'll say that I was very disappointed at myself on Friday. I had a few bad days, but today you've made me very, very happy. I want to talk about it over a nice dinner. You name the place; I'll call you tomorrow and make the reservations."

I always believed that with women, when in trouble, "Feed'em." Take her to an expensive restaurant that she could tell her girlfriends about.

Without pausing, I added, slow and jivey,

"And do me a big favor. I know you like to change around, but wear your hair the same as you had it on Friday. Put your face on perfectly again and wear the same scent. That's all been with me since Friday. That's not too much to ask, is it?"

She sounded just as subdued as she did when she first spoke. It was a very dry, "If I can."

I was still on punishment; she wasn't going to show me any enthusiasm. I wasn't to hear that pleasant sassiness in her voice, or see that room-brightening smile which I could see even over the telephone.

I understood, and I didn't allow it to dampen my joy.

The next day when I was at work, I would take out the picture, take a quick look at it, and again, just as quickly, turn it over to read "I love you." I still felt that rush.

The words are just symbols in the only language that I know. But when they're addressed to you, they elicit strong, wonderful feelings.

When I called her Thursday evening, I was expecting to spend the big bucks. I figured that this was to be a punishment meal. She kept the suspense going by not telling me the name of the restaurant. She said she had made the reservations in my name and all I had to do was pick her up at seven on Friday.

She looked stunning as she walked out to my car, but she didn't flash that "are you ready for dessert smile" that I was used to.

In the car, she sat so far away that she could easily lean out the other window. I got no smile and no, "hello sugah." But I sort of expected it, and I was prepared to be extra chipper for the both of us.

"Wow! You took my advice. You're looking very, very nice."

I received a chilly, "Thank you."

As chipper and jivey as I could be, I said,

"So babe, where to? What's it gonna be?

She said, "We won't be late; I want to go by your apartment and hear about any decisions you've made concerning us."

I thought that was an excellent idea. I figured I could warm up what had started out as a chilly evening, and my apartment was less than ten minutes away. I felt she was giving me the home court advantage.

Being a bachelor, I affectionately referred to my apartment as "the killing grounds." The Boys and I had this expression, "the dreadful work," we used concerning hounding women for sex. We would greet each other with, "The dreadful work must go on."

I felt now that I could run down my lines perfectly.

When we got in the apartment, I asked her if we had time for a quick, light drink. She said yes.

She had taken a seat in the chair, as opposed to being

by me on the sofa. I said,

"You're going to sit way over there?"

"Bobby, will you say what you have to say?"

"OK, give me a minute. This is very important to me."

It was awkward as hell. Me being on the sofa, and she being, what felt like, far, far away. I didn't like how the evening had started out. I had been pumped up for three days and this gamesmanship was not what I wanted. But, I didn't blame her; just for picking up a picture that should have remained face down.

Nevertheless, she had taken the initiative to say I love you first, and I really wanted to say something to let her know that I felt the same way. I wanted her to feel that wind gust of joy I had felt. So I dropped the little cute lines I had planned to say — game time was over. As I spoke, I was pausing between each phrase.

"Since Wednesday when I opened your letter... sitting right here where I am now... I've been thinking and thinking about something I could say to let you feel the joy I felt at that moment. And I'm sorry... I can't come up with anything."

She said nothing, just stared at me with those pretty eyes, although I did see a change in her face. She didn't smile, but her look was softer. You know what I mean — that pre-smile look.

I headed into my more jivey speech pattern, "Cyn, before I go on, if you don't mind, I would really like you to sit over here. Sit real close. When two people love each other that's what they do."

Bam! just like that, I had gotten it out, and I didn't give her time enough to say anything. I was patting the spot on the sofa while I said a begging-like, "Please."

She walked over slowly and sexy, I might add. She sat very close beside me, but it was too soon for me to try and get some sugah. I couldn't seal everything with a kiss, because she hadn't even smiled yet. As she sat down, I said,

"Let me show you something."

I took her picture out of my wallet.

"I got this laminated real thick. It seals in everything, so you won't be able to take it back."

Then I turned it over to the writing,

"This is real, real sweet. But, you're intuitive, you know I've felt this way for awhile. It started around Christmas, and I know I've shown it since then."

She had warmed up a little by now. She put her drink down, twisted her body, and with both hands on the back of my head, pulled my head toward hers. I thought she was finally about to give me some sugah, but she just drew us together forehead to forehead.

With her hands on my jaws, and looking me straight in the eyes, she said slowly, but emphatically,

"Why are you such a fumbler, bumbler?"

I couldn't say anything, because she added,

"You know... you're making it difficult for me to."

And she paused searching for the right words,

"To let myself go all out, give myself completely."

I said, "Why would you say that? You know how I feel. How I act toward you."

Then I quickly added, "Oh! I get it. You want an operator, a slick Chicago niggah."

"No! that's not what I'm saying at all."

Then she looked at me, waiting for me to respond. She had that expression that says, "You're supposed to be hip. Can't you see what I'm saying?"

Finally, I said, "Men have to protect their feelings too. And you are a Chicago girl. But, if you're saying that from now on, you want it to be me and you, an exclusive relationship, I would like that. Is that what you're saying?"

"Exactly! That's the only way it can be."

"Cyn, why did you have to put it like that? That sounds like an ultimatum or something. Can you say it sweeter?"

She said, "That's how I would like for us to be."

I replied lovingly, "And that's how I would love for us to be."

And we sealed it with a kiss.

I was feeling real happy. I told her,

"This is much better. You were real cold when you got in the car."

"You deserved it."

I was on a love high. So I pulled one of my impromptu stunts. The kind I can never forget, and it keeps that night and that scene in my mind forever. I said,

"Before we go to dinner; I want to write this."

I got a felt pen off the table, reached over and pulled her dress up on her thigh,

"Can't anybody see this," I said. I wrote "I love you, Bobby." And she really surprised me, "What if my daughter sees that?"

She sounded upset, and I was thinking, why didn't she say something when I started writing. She continued with, "She likes to sleep with me sometimes. I tell her all the time to not let little boys go under her dress."

I didn't know what to say because I thought I had been very romantic.

Cyn closed her eyes, sighed deeply for about a second. She opened her eyes, glared at me intently, and she said slowly and sweetly, "Now... lick it off!"

Talk about a quick, unpredictable, funny, sensual woman, Cyn was it. We were well-matched. I was fast with a quip, and she was just as fast.

While I was cracking up, she pulled her dress over her knees, and gave me a hug while saying,

"It's time for dinner. I like what you wrote."

I knew her stunt was just a sexy joke, and I had been forgiven for last Friday. So I said, "OK, babe. You know I mean it. Where's dinner gonna be?"

"Just go to Ribs and Bibs and hurry back."

"What! I thought I had to spend the big bucks tonight?"

"I couldn't think of any place expensive enough, but you'll get your chance."

"You're sure you don't want to go out."

"No. It's been a rough week at work, and you didn't help things out."

Last Friday was the last thing I wanted mentioned now, so I tried to be funny.

"You mean I took a shower and put on some clean drawers for nothing?"

She had taken off her shoes and grabbed the remote control, so I knew she was serious about not wanting to go out.

I wanted to assure her, without saying it outright, that it was me and her now. I was getting all other women out of my life.

"When you decide when and where you want to go, make it any day of the week and any time. I'm available, it's me and you, babe."

We, apparently, believed each other's proclamation of love. As you know, love is more than just saying you do. Enough months had passed where "what we said" and that love ritual of "what you do" had blended. So our being in love was very believable, and that was a stretch for me.

I know men are accused of telling women they love them to get what they want, but I always saw women as the ones just throwing around the expression of "I love you," especially in the days before the sexual revolution and the whole concept of the independent woman.

In the mid-seventies, women could be intimate with you without love being mentioned. In the old days, the "I love you" message to the man was that good girls screwed you because they loved you. For themselves it was, "I'm not a whore, respect me in the morning, and call me the next day."

When a guy in the mid-seventies called the next day, sometimes he was greeted with, "I had a very nice night, but don't read more into it than it really is."

It was real ego-adjusting times, and not the type of thing that guys would readily admit to, if they admitted it at all.

Anyway, it was an unforgettable week. I had no idea, at the time how much I would grow to love her. I wasn't too familiar with the expression "soulmate," and I didn't know that she would be the love of my life.

I knew that being with any good-looking woman, plus partying, equals good times, and good times were enough for me. But there's a level of joy beyond having a good time. Good times, plus love, equals happiness, and that was what lay ahead.

I never wanted to be in a heavy relationship with two boring people deeply in love, clinging pathetically to each other through some good, but too many bad times. I saw an airy love affair full of love stunts, love expressions, and challenges.

For a woman like Cyn, I knew to prepare myself for some drama and mystery and she didn't disappoint me. I sized up the future correctly and it was full steam ahead.

Monarch Butterfly Morning

gracefulness
fragility
feminality
pretty one
color of

oranges, licorice, and ivory.

nectareous
sun worshiper
wind rider
here and there

courtesan of wildflowers.

noiseless drifter
hoverer
floater
summer's child,

you've made this day but
everyday and everything is
    beautiful,

she said that she loves me.

A Man in Love

in Winter,
snowfalls were blinding, silent
but now I hear the soft pattering
of snow-flakes falling,

in Spring,
I feel vibrations from saplings
pushing their way through the
moistened black soil,

in Summer,
clouds are low, drifting, sunlit
and I overhear muffled-clunkings
of those swelling cumulus clouds
bumping each other,

in Autumn,
I see maple leaves turning brown
red, orange, and smiling
and hugging one another goodbye
right before leaping into a gale
prettily dying,

I see everything differently now,
I feel everything deeper because
I'm a man
effervescent, I'm a man blooming,
I'm a man in heat,
I'm a man in love.

Femininity

When Cynthia was by my side, she asked me often, "Why are you so good to me? Why do you love me so much?"

I loved hearing the questions, and I had a standard answer which I used like a refrain, "Because you're very feminine, the ultimate woman, quintessential female."

I said a little more sometimes, but in those technicolor days I didn't dwell too much on why I loved her. In those sweet times, I was too busy enjoying being with her. When a couple is deeply in love, there are a number of cliches they use to explain why. "We were just meant to be together," or "Ours is a match made in heaven." I thought my answer to Cyn was enough because it was, at the least, a little bit different.

Since those questions stay with me even today, I started analyzing some of the things about her that made her so unforgettable. I know it was a feminine stimulus, something awakening my senses that was sensual as well as sensuous. Everything in my consciousness and subconsciousness that attracted me to a woman was in collision with her femininity. So I'll begin with analyzing femininity beyond my curiosity about it in the past. First, saying that we had a very satisfying sexual life is too bourgeois and clinical. In an extended relationship, there is a standard of performance that I want from my woman. I expect to be, and I was, in effect, "pussy-whipped." But besides being lucky enough to be in that splendiferous state of being, what else?

I stated that Cyn was very feminine, and like most males, I'm aware of a few things about what that means. I know it's a gender-produced allurement that's a function of their design, so it's possessed by all females. I know it's rooted in eroticism, our love of physical beauty, and it's sometimes referred to as femaleness. Also, I'm fully aware that it's an essential element in the propagation of the species. But beyond those things, I'm hard pressed to put the attraction into words. Maybe it's not meant to be verbalized succinctly. Even in higher primates, some things are just meant to be felt and reacted to.

My bottom line in determining how far I was willing to go in a relationship was whether a woman was sweet or not. This is the essential ingredient of my simplest definition of femininity. However, I couldn't stay with that simple definition to explain a woman like Cynthia. Sweetness was just the first layer in a very complex appeal. I knew our first year that it was infatuation along with love. She was the prettiest girl I was ever involved with, but it was much more than that. Today I call her appeal "labyrinthic femininity." It means her femininity was complicated, intricate, involved, and many-layered. It's that maze or labyrinth that a man is confronted with when he seeks to totally understand a woman, and part of his excitement is in knowing that he never will.

Like most men, I've always observed women, but I've always been careful not to be caught staring. It's an innocent, fun, and exciting thing to do. I think it's hypocritical for some women to complain that they're being stared at as sex objects. They know they're in the gym and stay in those stores shopping because they're trying to catch a man. Or they simply want to look their best for the gawkers. Of course, girl-watching today is more than instinctual. It's like having an appreciation of art. It's admiring style and even pomposity. I've looked at a woman and wanted to stop and ask her, "Who does your hair? Where did you get those boots?" I want to compliment a woman on her sense of style because she has a look, a flair, I would like to see on my woman.

Like any other man, something indistinguishable and mysterious first attracts me to a woman. It's physical, but it's more than that because there are many fine and beautiful women I'm not attracted to. I was first attracted to Cynthia because she had a pretty face. It wasn't that sultry type of prettiness, but a classy, intelligent look. She looked soft, feline, and she had that feline grace of movement. She had a nice bustline, but height-wise she wasn't my type. She was shorter than the women I would hit on at the time. Being six-foot-three, I was drawn to taller women. But Cyn was tall enough, and she had that mysteriousness about her. It was strong enough to set the game in motion.

Why do I love her so much, and why can't I give her up? Today I'm analyzing her appeal as carefully as I can, and when I think of her I see variations of several women. She had this facility for easily moving in and out of opposites. Opposites like delicacy and wilfulness, sassing and assuaging, dependency and independence, and girlishness and womanliness. I saw her being one woman one day and another the next. And this is definitely a part of the answers I'm seeking.

I like feminine, costumery, pretty things on a woman. Cyn was the type who could feminize male things. Whatever she put on, the woman within would always shine through. I had a thick, solid-gold, nugget ring that I wore on my pinky. One night Cyn tried it on her middle finger. Instantly, the ruggedness of the ring just disappeared, and it looked so pretty on her finger. I didn't wear it again; I gave it to her that same night.

Because society puts women on display, they probably have an earlier awareness of their best features, what it is about them that appeals to men the most. And they seem to have this curiosity about their overall effect on a man. One evening Cyn asked me if infatuation was a part of my love for her. Before I gave an answer, I was thinking, "Infatuation! Damn! How cocky can a woman be? I guess it's my job to verify some line other guys had dropped on her over the years." My answer to her was, "Don't get too cocky about it, but sure, I'm very much fascinated and infatuated by you."

And quickly she asked, "Why?"

"Baby! You're the ultimate woman, quintessential female."

"Are you ever going to break that down?"

She knew I was the type of guy who didn't have to know the answer to give an answer. I was going to lie or say something that at least had some element of truth in it. One time she summed up my approach to things by saying, "You know baby, at least you try to be deep." (She was sweet and complimentary like that.)

Anyway, she asked me to write her a letter, so I said, "Sure, I'll write you a letter. But for right now, it has something to do with your natural femininity. Plus, all of the soft tricks and games you use to hold on to me."

"Okay Bobby, whatever. But be more serious in the letter."

I was serious. Those soft tricks and games were a good show and very entertaining. They were an outlet for her to express herself in different ways to a lover that she knew was observant and appreciative of feminine wiles.

Cyn was very intelligent, and I really like intelligent women. We all look up to any person who manifests a high mental capacity, but a lot of times when a guy tells a woman that he likes her for her mind, she thinks he's running down a line. Maybe sometimes, but attractiveness is very complex. It's been a long time since "Lucy" walked the misty, fertile plains of prehistoric Africa. Today a woman's appeal is based on many things that are addendums to our basic instincts. Intelligence is one of them, and it has its own power of attraction. Intelligence is an aura-enhancing of whatever else a woman brings to the table. I can't explain it, but it's definitely sexual. When I met Cyn and looked into her eyes, I saw the look of intelligence. It's as distinctive as the look of joy or irritation. It accounts for a woman's feminine qualities such as graciousness, sensitivity, subtleness, vulnerability, and capriciousness, but also a sassy decisiveness.

It's a false perception that an intelligent, educated woman is an unskilled laborer between the sheets. Just because a woman is eloquent, well-read, analytical, and more often than not, stylish, it doesn't impede her ability to be what every man wants, which is a whore in bed (an irrepressive and sensual lover). Actually, it's the quick contrast from her normal sophisticated and, cultured persona to a natural woman in heat that's so appealing. And this woman is oneup on women who rely mainly on sexuality to entice and hold on to a man, because when the bed is made, the intelligent woman's show is not over. Personally, I couldn't have a relationship over a period of time with a woman who isn't intelligent, well-read, opinionated, proud of her heritage, has a social conscience, is spiritual, and funny. Of course, Cyn was all of these.

My first conversation with Cynthia convinced me that she was the type of city girl I had wanted to meet. She was urbane and sophisticated, but she also had that grassroots appeal. A great part of any woman's femininity is the sound of her voice and her level of articulation. When I was growing up down South, we characterized a certain manner of speaking as being northern or "talking proper." Cynthia had that polished manner of speaking. But, as with most things about her, she was very versatile. Her speech pattern was functional, and she was multi-dialectal. When necessary, she was able to use professional jargon, black slang, or Chicago hipness. She didn't use profanity as a regular part of her speech, but she did use it for emphasis sometimes if she was really pissed off.

Like many women, Cyn used being well-read, her fluency, and overall intelligence as a part of her natural charm and sensuality. I see these qualities as part of the manipulative tools a sophisticated woman carries in her arsenal, and I don't mean manipulative in a negative sense. They're attributes that make a woman more interesting. Cyn's appeal could be classy or earthy; it depended on her mood and what she wanted to project at a particular time.

Without a doubt, my feelings for Cynthia were deepened by my knowledge of how she felt about herself and for me. She really loved me. She said it, showed it, and I could feel it. I knew she would do anything for me, and she was always there for me, as the cliche goes. But it was one important thing she didn't do that a lot of women make a big mistake in doing. She didn't love me more than she loved herself. When you do that you're disrespecting yourself and you're inviting unhappiness for yourself. We both understood that we couldn't just do anything to the other; we couldn't just say anything. Loving and respecting ourselves was the foundation which warded off treatment that eventually leads to unhappiness. This was the other side of the equation, besides our not living together, that sustained our high level of romanticism and our long years of happiness

The desire to know women is a part of every man's makeup, and I guess women feel the same way about men. I've always imagined that women actually discussed ways to put the concept of femininity into action. I imagined them networking approaches aimed to blow our weak, male creatures minds. As a result, I look at femininity the same way I look at an actress in a predictable scene. I'm watching to see how she's going to pull it off. Cyn was very subtle in manipulating the feminine mystique, and she was consistently unpretentious. I felt as though it was natural; she was showing me something real. But even if she wasn't, I enjoyed the performance.

Cyn had many ways to say "I love you" through body language and touch. It was natural, and maybe on the surface not much different from what other women do: leaning her head on my shoulder, my chest, brushing against me, holding my hand, or throwing kisses. But this body language and touching done in unison with those pretty eyes and her sultry presence, created an enclosed space. A space where there was just the two of us, whether we were at a play, in a mall, in the Loop, or actually alone.

I used to call Cyn "pretty lady" all the time, and I was first attracted to her as another pretty face. But it was an attraction from a mature man's viewpoint, not like a fifth-grader who is flipping for the prettiest little girl in his class, or even a teenager who is fascinated with the best-looking girl in his neighborhood. In deference to attractive, good looking, or pretty women, they're a dime a dozen. And I don't mean that negatively because I have a fascination for them. But they're on every other street corner, so I always search for what else they have going for them.

I moved with a deliberate controlled speed after being attracted to Cynthia. If I had known her essence, that well of kindness behind those pretty eyes, I would have moved with a desperate speed. But to know a person takes time. It was time that taught me all of those wonderful things about her such as her spirituality, great capacity for giving and receiving love, ability to share, sense of loyalty, compassion for others, and the way she made me feel as a man, as her man. These are the reasons, so much more than the way she looked, that I loved her so much. And why in this black early morning, I am compelled to write about her.

I wanted to say these things first before I talked further about my pretty lady. The sociologist who said a passionate lover is fascinated by every aspect of the one he loves was right on the money. Every feminine thing about her becomes another weapon in her arsenal. In my mind's eye, I'm still looking at Cynthia, and I see all of those things like her smile, her hair, her lips, and her body that I had claimed as my own. Maybe that's all that femininity is, something you see about her, and something you feel about her.

Today I still see her beautiful eyes burning through the marrow of my bashfulness. Like most women, she really knew how to use her second voice. That's a pet term I used for her communicating with her eyes. I liked to ask her in a whisper, "Hey babe, tell me something sweet with your second voice?" It was something else about her that imprinted me to her. In a stare, a glance, or a sweep of her eyes she told me what she wanted me to know. I saw her eyes moisten in spiritual fervor and sparkle with joy and laughter. She could sweep with the look of love, or summon with a look of lust. They were all naturally and easily done.

A female is something soft, smooth, and tressed.

Like most men, I consider a woman's hair a very important element of her femininity. It can be long or short, but it always gives her a different persona, sometimes soft, hard, chic, or professional. I think a hairstyle definitely gives a clue to a woman's social class and what she's about. Cyn considered her hair to be one of her best features, and she spent a lot of money and time making sure it looked good. I really loved her hair, too; it was one of the things that attracted me to her. Naturally, as her lover man, I believed I had the right to decide which style looked best on her. Her reply to that was, "You got to be crazy." But I knew she liked my great interest in her hairstyles, and if I raved enough about one, she kept it for awhile. A woman's haircut can make a splendid date. It stays on a guy's mind as much as a sharp outfit.

I used to drive Cyn all the way to the near-north side to get her hair done. I would drop her off and go back later to pick her up. I got tired of driving that far, so I volunteered to pay for her to get her hair done by this so-called "Egyptian artist" who was skilled at doing black women's hair. It included a perm, cut, and styling. After that, I stopped complaining about driving her to get her hair done as long as I didn't have to pay that unbelievable price for simply rearranging hair strands. Of course, sometimes I ended up driving her a long way and paying to get it done too. There's one inescapable fact about having a fine, good-looking woman. They're like a slot machine — you have to put some money in them.

Cyn was feminine to the core. She had very beautiful hands, too. I would lift her hand by placing my hand, face up, under hers. I just admired its slightness, her long slender fingers, and painted natural nails. I always let her know in a whisper how I felt about her hands because the color was even, and they were beautiful, soft, and erogenous. But it was her lips that I stared at while she slept. They always reminded me of how beautiful black women's lips are. Cyn's were sculptured, full, nubian, and expressive. They looked as though they were chiseled specifically to be magnetic, sensual, and admired, but to say nothing.

I'm not going to be able to give a definitive answer to Cyn's question of why I loved her so much, nor can I fully answer my own questions. I can only give bits and pieces about her femininity and my undying love. I know that in order to love any woman, a man has to be capable of loving and appreciating women. It's a part of our makeup given to us by our Creator. According to Genesis, woman was made from the rib of man so that man would not have to be alone. How can any man not honor this gift from God?

I always realized that I was living my romantic fantasy by loving Cynthia and being loved by her. All of us are actors in our own love stories, and they're just as real as those in romantic novels and what comes out of Hollywood. As far as beautiful women are concerned, they're virtually everywhere. And what a beautiful woman is to a man, at least his woman, shouldn't be dictated by Hollywood or the fashion industry. I guess it's no great harm to get caught up in the hype of women promoted as goddesses by Hollywood, television, and record companies, but a man shouldn't forget that his woman is a queen, exciting, and very beautiful too.

I'm back to my only answer. I want to be original and deep, but I really can't think of anything definitive to say to answer my own questions. I picked up this statement from somewhere, I used it then, and I'll use it now like a refrain. Maybe it's the simple and definitive answer that says everything. I loved her so much and I can't give her up because she was the ultimate woman, the quintessential female... and I believe this.

Female

Something soft
something sinewy

something tressed
something glabrous

something naive
something labyrinthine

something indifferent
something in heat

something huggable
something breakable

something beautiful
something maternal

something lovable
something completing

Something Female.

Labyrinthic Femininity

The Final Frontier?

Some men say it's space while
other men say the ocean depths.

All perceptive men know it's
    a woman.

    She's
unfathomable, but fulfilling,

    unconquerable
through times of stoning,
inquisitions and scarlet letters.

    She's that
mysterious realm of a being
feared, hated, pursued, loved,
contagious, and addicting.

    The same
species, the same gender,
but they're all one of a kind.

    Contrastable
like tints of the color blue,
azurine, berylline, sapphirine,
turquoise, and robin's-egg-blue.

    She's
changeable, not interchangeable.

They're
multifarious like wildflowers,
black-eyed susans
water lilies
african violets
oxeye daisies and goldenrods.

Distinct natures
feel, looks, carnality, sighs
moans, essence, illusoriness.

Although
sprayed with the same cologne
their scents are heterogeneous.

Thankfully,
she's always more woman than
what the last man knew of her.

And her femaleness
her flavor, unforgettableness,
and that beauty possessed by
one woman,

maybe liken, analogous, and is
sometimes fondly reminiscent,
but it is never the same as in
another woman.

Pretty Woman

Since I can remember,
been drawn to pretty things,
they make us feel good.

Something pretty,
is a stallion at full gallop,
Willie Mays at full gallop,
a burgundy, phaeton roadster.

Something pretty,
an emerald pond full of bowl
shaped leaves on tiny stalks
and swaying above in
honeysuckle-scented southern
summer breezes are scores of
pale-yellow American Lotuses
but nevertheless,

there's something even prettier.

It's a pretty woman and
the look that makes her pretty
is being in love
so, every woman who is in love

is a pretty woman

because being in love radiates
that exact, shining, beautiful
glow of a woman with child and
as everybody knows, certainly
every man,
nothing is prettier than that!

Mercuriality

One minute she's a little girl,
the next minute, she's a woman
        She can
look sweet and unsophisticated
if she wants to, and glamorous
hot and steamy if it suits her.

        One night
she's possessive and obsessive,
but she's as aloof as a pretty
Burmese cat just the following
        evening.

        Most of the times
I'm her mentor, older, wiser
        and
she leans very heavily on me,

        but she's
my caring nurse if I am sick,
she's my thoughtful therapist
        when I'm floundering.

        One week
I feel she totally belongs to
me but the next week she only
        belongs to herself,

        and
I'm forever changing a lot too,
one minute I love her and
the next, I love her much more.

Butterfly Feminist

There's a good percentage of men who view feminism as the antithesis of femininity, but I'm not one of them. Of course, I have a comedic side about feminism that has me longing for the "good old days," but my serious side views the feminist movement the same way I view the civil rights movement, which I was a part of. A relationship just may be a microcosm of the so-called war between the sexes, and the "Boys" have always said that it will be A over B, or B over A. There's no such thing as A and B together. It is a consensus among men that women really love a take-charge guy. I would be lying if I said I didn't see an element of truth in these statements. Still, my goal with Cyn was not to try and dominate her. Whether it was totally true or not, I saw myself as a good man. I believed that Cyn would recognize me as a good man, and she would respond to me positively.

Even if I ask her, I'm really not that interested in a woman's past relationships. It was Cyn and I now, and things were going to be different and better. I was thankful for her growth, and Cyn was the woman she presented to me. I knew that Cynthia very well. Still, I can only speak for her on the things she clearly articulated at the time. I'll speak mostly from my observations about her feminist impulses within our relationship. I can say for certain that she didn't play the role of the "permanent victim." Neither did she elevate women, as a whole, to the status of the "noble gender" which was never at fault.

It might be chauvinistic for me to put it this way, but since I like to name things, I'm going to call her a "butterfly feminist." This term does not apply to political or economic rights, but feminism within a relationship. A woman affirming her rights as an equal partner through teaching and deprogramming. Hers was a soft sell, but not the flirtatious batting of the eyes and a sweeter-than-sweet voice saying, "You're the man! Please treat lil' old me right."

It was more like she looked me straight in the eyes and said, "We love each other. That means respecting my views and wishes. There are some things about me, and our relationship that you may not be attuned to at times. I'll tell you as deliberately and as rationally as I can about them, and I expect you to make a sincere effort to get your shit together if you value this relationship."

That was Cyn. That was how she ran things down, and it was basically the same as my approach. We were constantly articulating our particular viewpoints.

There's such a thing as looking sweet. A woman can project a girlishness; a softness seen in innocent little girls that makes them kissable and huggable, like fluffy animal toys. They're able to bring out that paternal urge that men show toward "Daddy's little girl." The simple joy of walking along holding his daughter's hand, showing her the world, protecting her from the world, and buying her pretty things. I don't have a daughter, but I've always wanted one, and this is the way I imagined it would be.

Some of the feelings I had for Cyn were a lot like the feelings I probably would have felt for a daughter. Also, she reflected how I felt about my mother, because I saw Cyn as a nurturing mother. A man wants to protect his woman as if she's still a little girl, and strangely, many women reject this feeling. I felt protective about Cynthia, but there must have been something lost in the translation of my feelings, or something wrong about the way I acted on them. Her father was killed in a robbery when she was in college. That was about seven years before we started dating. There were times she would say to me "My daddy is dead, I don't need another daddy." At first, it caught me off guard because I didn't know what she meant. But I knew that a woman can become more upset about the man in her relationship acting like he's her daddy than a man would be about a woman acting like she's his mother.

One of the things Cyn stressed was to be aware of, and to guard against, latent paternalism. She distinctly disliked me, in her words, "playing daddy." I didn't see myself as being bossy or wanting to be anybody's daddy. I never totally reconciled to the idea that I sometimes acted that way to her. But in fairness, there may have been some paternalism that popped up every once in a while in my approach to things. Maybe because I was older, or maybe it's just a male thing. Either way it was a natural instinct and inadvertent.

I don't think ours was a rare case. Apparently, many grown women believe that there's latent paternalism in a lot of relationships, and we men can take this daddy thing too far. Cyn stressed that it was paternalism, as opposed to chauvinism, because she was really hard on a real chauvinist. She saw a staunch male chauvinist as an ignorant man who was sometimes amusing, but definitely had problems. She believed that any chauvinist with power over women was dangerous. On the other hand, she felt that loving and good intentions were a part of my paternalism, and I simply had to be straightened out every once in a while. Most black women like to use the phrase, "I had to get him told."

So I learned that sweetness, or as Muddy Waters put it in a song, "Ways Like a Baby Child," doesn't give a boyfriend the authority of a daddy. Sweetness and perceived naivete are just natural parts of some women's appeal, but to act girlish should not be confused with being a girl. A girl is someone a man has to take by the hand and guide where he wants her to go while interpreting her reality of the world.

Cyn was telling me that she knew where she was going, and she was intelligent enough to deal with the complexities of life. She wanted me to recognize that she was a professional, serious about her work, confident in making decisions in raising her family, and she was doing a pretty good job. I really felt this way all along, but it's something that a man should verbalize occasionally.

Of course, I had to explore this daddy thing a little more, "OK Cyn, let me get this perfectly clear. First, I'm not trying to be a daddy, but are you saying you don't expect the man in your life to protect you?"

"In general, sure."

"All right, I get the picture. A boyfriend is supposed to be like a bodyguard: walk you to the door, make sure you get in safely, and risk his life protecting you from the big, bad city, but this doesn't make him your boss. Also, you don't need him to be acting like a watch-dog daddy, protecting you from men in general, unless the guy is persistently obnoxious. But most of all, if it's a good-looking guy who merely wants to get under your skirt, you alone reserve the right to resolve that problem, right?"

"You know Bobby, you really have a keen insight into your role. I couldn't have put it better myself."

The moral to this little predicament was very clear. A grown woman does not want a man in her life other than her father playing daddy… that is… unless he's a "sugar daddy."

I'm calling Cynthia a "butterfly feminist" because she stood up for herself as a woman in her own gracious way. I was a supporter and an advisor to her about things if asked, but she made the final decisions. There was another small idiosyncrasy about me that got on her nerves. I recall her telling me that I was always right. She meant that I thought and argued as though I were always right. One day the truth of her assertion hit me. I'm argumentative by nature. I love a good debate and an analysis of a situation. But again, I felt I was right because I was older and male. On occasions I would say, "You know, Babe, you've got to get over that penis envy thing." And then I would grab between my crotch and say, "This gives me the authority to decide what's right and what's wrong."

I wonder how many other guys out there have pulled off that scene. Probably a lot. I didn't really, believe it, but it was fun to do. When I thought seriously about what Cyn had said, I had to concede that I did argue to win, right or wrong. I was right many times, but not all of the time. But I love pontificating; it's the teacher in me.

It also took me a while to pick up on several very important differences when listening and conversing with a woman as opposed to a man. This time she didn't say anything at all to me about the particular situation. It was away to teach me a lesson by leaving the situation alone. Cyn would talk to me about problems on the job or at home. I assumed she was asking me how I would go about solving the problems. I ran off several ways that I saw as the best ways to deal with the situations. Sometimes I would critique the way she handled the situation. It was either too soft or too indecisive. You know, a man running down how a man would go about solving the problem.

The result was she just stopped talking to me about any problems. But I could hear her on the telephone talking to girlfriends about problems at work or at home. It bothered me a little, but I didn't want to ask her why she didn't confide in me anymore. I let it go for awhile. Soon it occurred to me that Cyn was doing most of the talking. The girlfriend was listening and would occasionally give a short opinion. I arrived at the right conclusion, even though I came through the chauvinist route.

"I see, she's not interested in me solving the problem. She just want somebody to sit, listen, and boo-hoo with her about it." I figured she wanted me to attend these "pity parties" that women like to engage in. But her turning me off taught me a lesson. She didn't need me to validate her actions. She wanted me to listen sometimes without comment. Sometimes through just her talking, she could find a solution. After all, what did I know about operating in the corporate world? She had female and male friends she could go to lunch with to talk about how to proceed. My job was to be a sympathetic listener and to be there for her. That's probably all that women ask of their men sometimes, so I tried to be a more patient and sympathetic listener.

Cyn would tell me some things about herself concerning old boyfriends because she knew I was not silly enough to be jealous about things that happened long before I knew her. I just had to be careful not to be judgmental, and I was to never bring up something she had confided to me, in an argument, for reasons of my own at a later time. Of course, I did this a few times earlier on in our relationship, but after going through the long process of rebuilding trust, I learned my lesson.

I'm tempted to make myself appear as though I was an enlightened, chauvinist-free male back in those days. But to be truthful, I didn't share any real secret, with Cyn because she was a woman. And I really believed that one of the most useless statements to tell a woman was, "I'm gonna tell you this, but I want it to be kept strictly confidential." In my mind, on that same night she would get on the phone and tell a girlfriend the secret and soon the secret would be going from girlfriend to girlfriend like a chain letter.

One of the advantages men expected from a true feminist was to see less tears. Maybe it's a generalization, but it seems that women are always crying about something happening in their lives, and most guys believed that crying was used as a ploy to elicit sympathy on many occasions. Our relationship was peppered with a lot of little predicaments, but it was virtually devoid of tears. Even a butterfly feminist didn't cry about life situations; she took it like a man. On a personal level, it was only one time right after Cyn had turned thirty that I may have been responsible for her crying. It was a time when I could have exclaimed, "So! You're not so tough after all." But it didn't turn out that way.

I was clowning around and I told Cyn that she was over the hill, she didn't have it anymore, and then she broke. She started crying loud and hard. I was stunned. "Wait! Don't do that, I'm sorry. I was just joking." It was in our fourth year of being together. I knew that she was soft-hearted, but this was unexpected. Sometimes she was wet-eyed when she and her daughter had gotten into an argument. But I hadn't made her shed a single tear, unless she had been laughing too hard. My heart melted; my big mouth had made my baby cry. I struggled to apologize, but didn't have the words to let her know I didn't mean what I had said. I should have known never to tell a woman who had been told all of her life that she was cute, that she was over the hill. And especially, right after she turned thirty. By the third day of my many heartfelt apologies and gestures of love, she said, "Look, it's OK. You just go too far sometimes, but don't feel bad about it anymore. It was one of those things that happened after I couldn't button my pants that morning, and I looked in the mirror at how fat my face had gotten."

"What! You knew I was just joking, but you let me grovel and feel bad over something that wasn't entirely my fault."

"You told me a woman's tears didn't mean a damn thing to you."

"I can't believe this. You let me go through changes for three long days just because you picked up a little weight?"

I saw this as an opening for me to make up some for

messing up, so I hugged her while rapping sweetly, "Baby you're looking better than ever. You know the brothers don't like that skinny model type. When I'm in bed to take care of some serious business, I don't want to play that game 'find the woman.' I like my barbeque ribs and my woman with some meat on 'em."

Like the typical feminist, she took advantage of my sweetness by squeezing me back and whispering much sweeter, "So you're gonna buy me some new clothes?"

"Ain't this a bitch. I'm trying to console you, and you're trying to take advantage of it."

She continued triumphantly, "You know baby you sho' can beg. I don't know whether I want a man to love me that much. You won't kill me if I try to leave?"

I was genuinely pissed off. "This shit ain't funny Cyn. I had three bad days."

"Babe, you really, really know how to stroke a woman's vanity."

"You mean I really know how to stroke."

"That too, baby."

She may have been playing the guilt trip game, and the how-much-does-he-love-me game, but in a land that worships youth, I had struck an untimely note. Still, it was really just like she had said. Her crying was from a combination of things and my big mouth.

Cyn's brand of feminism was great to build a strong relationship with. I couldn't completely dominate her even if I had wanted to, because she had no desire to simply be the extension of a man. Even though she was in love with me, she knew she could get another man in spite of my persistent campaign to convince her that I was the best. But I loved her self-confidence and independent spirit because it allowed me to be myself.

I'm aware that I have some views that alienate women sometimes. But saying them is a good habit of mine that's left over from the honest, straightforward relationship I had with Cynthia. We expected each other to give our opinions on relationships. So I'm saying, because Cyn wasn't the pitiful-type woman sitting around waiting on a man to make her happy, it took a lot of pressure off of me. It's not that I totally disliked being depended and leaned on, but some women take this too far. Their happiness is like a third job and double-overtime for a man. They don't really want a man; they want a court jester. Some guy to break into a soft-shoe tap dance to cheer them up when they're down, and one of the reasons they're always down is they have no other interests in life other than their man. Everybody knows that a great part of a relationship is attempting to make each other happy and that there's a joy in giving. But in my opinion, too many women expect a man to make them happy, and it's asking too much for one person to make another happy by making themselves unhappy.

I worked very hard helping to keep our relationship fresh and strong, but Cyn didn't require every ounce of me. She knew that I needed other outlets for my happiness, and this made our relationship less of a job and more of an adventure. So fortunately, I didn't have the problem of making myself unhappy to make Cindy happy. Cyn was a woman of varied interests: she was an activist, involved in her sorority, in a social club, and job-related organizations, involved in activities with her family, and worked in the service of the Lord. She had a lot of friends and acquaintances of all ages, races, and ethnic groups, both men and women. She made friends easily, and she kept expanding her list.

After the early years of mental jousting, our relationship enjoyed long periods of near-perfect peace. To a great degree, this was due to her articulating her positions on relationship issues, what she wanted, didn't like, liked, and what we could compromise on. Her style wasn't nagging nor adversarial. But her style was forceful enough for me to see her as an equal.

Because of the occasional irrationality of being politically correct these days, I had reservations about using the term "butterfly feminist." I thought that some feminists might view me as a male trying to dilute the aggressiveness inherent in the term "feminist." I had thought about naming the chapter, "Strong Black Woman." Cynthia was a descendant of strong black women like Harriet Tubman, Sojouner Truth, and thousands upon thousands of nameless female slaves who fought for their very humanity in a life and death struggle. I concluded that if I diluted anything in using the term feminist, it was the historical activist tradition of the strong black woman.

Today, it's my understanding that "feminist" is a universal and unifying term, and Cyn accepted my recognizing her as a feminist. Nevertheless, because of her finesse, and her pleasing, sweet disposition, I had no other choice but to call her something delicate, something pretty... a butterfly feminist.

The Scent of Her Hair

When
I place my face against hers I'm
feeling all that she is, I can't
get any closer, I'm inhaling the
scent of her hair, and it's that
scent of an ancient beauty,

a natural woman
her almond face is reflecting in
the Nile, in a clear stream deep
in the African rain forest.

I want to get closer
I'm pressing my face against her
face, rolling her earlobe around
on my wet tongue, my exhaling is
echoing in her ear.

She's
a natural woman, natural beauty,
the scent of her hair is racing
through my nostrils smelling of
incense wood
jasmine, lanolin, and coconut oil.

I'm imprinted
I can find her anywhere because
her body belongs to me,
she's my natural woman and she's
a natural beauty.

In My Touch

Knowing her touch,
how it felt, what it said,
I wanted
to say I love you too and
I did.

It was in my grip when
I was holding her hand,
in the soft pressure
when I touched her face,

in my carefulness while I
was scratching her head,
in my fingers when
I shampooed her hair,
in my gentleness when
I was washing her back,

in my fondle on her fanny
when she passed by me,
in my rub on her tummy
when she was cramping,

in the brush of my lips
when I kissed her body,
in my hugging when it was
thundering and lightning,
in my caressing when
she was scared or down,
and it
was anytime, when she
just needed me to hold her.

Chauvinist of Sorts

I have a lot of time on my hands these days, and Cynthia and our relationship never leaves my head. I talk to her mother on the phone often, sometimes for hours. Sometimes she talks about when Cynthia was a little girl, and about their family as she grew up. They're delightful stories, a side of Cyn I never knew. Some of the things my mother-in-law reveals give me insight as to why Cyn reacted to me so favorably.

Since a relationship involves two people acting and reacting to each other, I started to analyze myself. It's helpful for me to recall incidents in my early life that helped shape my views on women and relationships. I know these views along with my adult views have something to do with my feelings toward Cyn.

I was in my early thirties when I became a bachelor again. I know it's not just me. A lot of men don't know much about women until they reach thirty. By thirty, men have played the game long enough to understand a woman's needs better.

I brought some theories and social practices about a relationship when I met Cyn, but they were not written in stone. Thankfully, they were still evolving. I believe the happiness we shared was partly the result of this evolving and my willingness to compromise.

I've always taken a lot of pride in my ability to get along with people. It's a family trait that my four brothers and I inherited from our father, but like everything else, this trait has some complexity.

A lot of guys can get along very well with other men. They can be a popular man's man, but these same men can have problems getting along with women. Sometimes it's all women, and other times it's just women with whom they become emotionally involved.

I think some men and women take this "war between the sexes" far too seriously. Maybe society should stop using that phrase, because it's really not a war. A relationship is a game at the most, and I believe a person who really considers the opposite sex an enemy has a problem.

I got along with Cynthia very well, and we could have been friends if not lovers. Ours wasn't a stormy relationship, but it was unpredictable and spicy. I've already penned her a butterfly feminist, and I know I'm a chauvinist of sorts, so I wondered whether that clash is what made us get along so well. After some thought, I believe that blending of philosophies and wills played a great part in our happiness.

How I saw myself as a chauvinist, and what Cyn told me about my chauvinism were two distinct viewpoints. I always referred to myself as a male chauvinist bull as opposed to a male chauvinist pig. By adding the word "bull," I felt that I was turning a label used by feminists as a putdown into something macho and acceptable.

One night I was ranting and raving about women when Cyn pinned her own chauvinist label on me. She had gotten disgusted with me running off at the mouth. After I declared myself a male chauvinist bull, she said, "Bob, shut up! You're a teddy bear. You just TALK shit."

Cyn didn't combine teddy bear and chauvinist into a general description of me; she just said, "teddy bear." Today, I'm giving myself the label "teddy bear chauvinist" because I believe that's what she meant, and that's the way she felt about me. She didn't like staunch male chauvinists, and she didn't see me as one, no matter how much smack I talked. Apparently, she was defining the difference between a chauvinist bull and a teddy bear chauvinist. I didn't act stupidly for the most part; I just ran off my mouth stupidly a lot of times.

I was very much aware of the balancing act men needed to perform to appeal to women. I believed in mixing a little sweetness with a little roguishness. I always wanted women to consider me a good, decent man, but I found out early that the idea of a good man is a concept subject to various interpretations by different women. Also, I found that the good in a good man didn't necessarily mean good in the normal sense of being morally excellent, virtuous, or righteous. Most so-called "ladies men" have none of those qualities, but they have a lot of women. I wasted most of my teenage years trying to be a good man in the righteous sense, and women saw me as inflicted with terminal slowness. As I added more dog to my act, the more successful I became with women.

When I analyze my makeup and philosophy about relationships, I'm reminded again about how things are always more complicated than simple. For instance, I have said that I'm always looking for a woman who's sweet, but even that statement calls for a little more explanation.

A number of things can be very misleading about what sweetness means in a woman; often things like sweetness are seen as shyness, meekness, naivete, or inexperience. A woman can be the complete opposite of all of these traits and still be sweet.

Cyn was assertive in many ways, but she was still a sweet woman. She was hip, logical, and experienced, and that was what I was looking for.

An experienced woman is not one that sleeps around

indiscriminately, but a woman who has had her share of boyfriends and maybe a husband, as men have had their share of girlfriends and maybe a wife.

So I was happy that we were both at similar stages in life. She had come to the table bringing some lost love, some heartbreak, but willing to leave that baggage behind. Both of us were ready to build on the past and not be crippled by it.

We moved cautiously, but after a period of time we were ready to open up our hearts. She brought the excitement that I had wanted and needed in a relationship.

My early experiences led me to really fall for a woman like Cyn because she was kind and good-natured. She was opinionated and argumentative in an entertaining way, but that doesn't mean that she couldn't and didn't come out of a hell-raising, "sapphire bag" every once in a while.

I guess I should explain the term "sapphire bag," because even though it might be a black expression, it is somewhat outdated. It pertains to the wife of Kingfish on the radio (and later television show) "Amos and Andy." Sapphire was hell-raising, bossy, and always doing what the brothers like to refer to as "castrating a man." Along with the rest of the brothers in my generation, I've always talked about an evil, argumentative woman as being a sapphire.

This was the type of woman I would never get deeply involved with. A man hasn't been dressed-down and cursed-out properly and efficiently until he's pissed off a real get-down-in-the-gutter, gut-bucket, sapphire. Until then, he only thinks he's been cursed out.

Most sisters can come out of a sapphire bag to a certain extent, especially if the situation called for it. But I dislike a woman who always has an attitude and is just mean-spirited in general. Cyn's put-down approach was more of an educated woman with a good command of the language — that sophisticated, quick wit with its satire and sarcasm really cuts through a man. That verbal advantage and satirical assault that sophisticated women use on some men is the reason why a lot of frustrated guys end up losing their cool and get physical and violent with women. Of course, my response was never physical.

They say that a man's idea of a woman is partly shaped by his relationship with his mama — a woman who would feed him, put clothes on his back, money in his pocket, and give him that mother's love, no matter how sorry a son he is. My mama really doted on her five boys, and we were good sons because of it. We could do no wrong, and my daddy could do no right.

My mama nagging my daddy triggered my first aversion to a hell-raising woman. At the time, I thought it was really rough, but now I know that I was reacting with a kid's perception. Upon reflection, I see a relatively calm household, because my parents didn't drink or smoke around the house, nor did they curse in general.

Looking back, I can see my mother fighting for dignity and self-respect in a male-dominated house, as well as outside of the house. Strangely, whatever her struggle really was, it didn't seem to bother my daddy.

In general, married men have conveyed the impression that marriage is hell, and nagging was just the way wives were. As a teenager sitting in the barber shop listening to grown men, I believed in that picture of women they were painting. Still, in my teens it was more funny than anything else.

Daddy wasn't the shopper around the house, and one day he came back from the store with a head of lettuce when my mother had asked him to get some cabbage. Man, talking about a sapphire tongue-lashing. It lasted about an hour.

Daddy just cooled-out reading the paper, but I had to reach down to see whether I still had some balls. I was definitely thinking, "I really love my mama, but ain't no way in hell for me to get involved with a woman who raised that much cain."

But my mama was sweet and really loved her boys. Sometimes she took our sides, even later when we were married and in the wrong.

One time during my first marriage on a Thanksgiving holiday, all of the men were in one room, and the daughter-in-laws and my first cousins were in the back room talking. As I passed by the room, I heard one of the women say, "Yeah! They can't do no wrong. Mrs. Gamble think 'dem boys' are a piece of Jesus."

That was followed by a lot of laughter and expressions of agreement. I was pissed and thought, "These women got nerve to talk about my mama, the sweetest woman in the world."

I guess that's why girlfriends were always screaming, "I ain't yo Mama!" I say that a woman treating a man as caring and sweet as his mama did is really showing her love for him, and this type of thinking makes me what many women are in denial about — I was a "mama-made chauvinist." Many of the women that complain about male chauvinism actually help to turn their sons into one. Any "catching hell" daughter-in-law will confirm that I'm right.

My mama was a remarkable woman in many ways, but she may have been, justly or unjustly, my first aversion to a real bossy woman. Of course, now I realize that the term "bossy woman" was one of those doublestandard terms used negatively against women at the time. For men, it was called "being assertive," which was a positive trait. My socalled bossy mama was the driving force in making sure that my four brothers and I all stood up like men and finished college. She told us we could be anything we wanted to be and she taught by example.

Amelia J. Gamble was some lady. She enrolled in college and graduated when she was in her thirties. At the time, she had four boys and was pregnant with my youngest brother. We were in high school and sort of bewildered by her — because she was in college at that age, and also because she was pregnant. Later, we realized what an unusual woman she was. When we went to college, we realized what a difficult thing it was for her to do. Still, at the time I accepted aggressiveness as a negative trait in a woman. Maybe as a result, I've always been in this frantic search for a quiet, sweet woman.

I loved my job; it brought me a lot of satisfaction, but happiness was having somebody and being in love. My relationship with Cyn was always on my mind. I know there's some good and bad in every relationship, but I expected the good to establish a dynasty. I wasn't going to be in an extended love affair with the bad. After all, a woman ain't the Chicago Cubs.

I didn't expect more from the relationship than what I could bring, and I believe I brought a lot of good. I'm a talker, a bullshitter, and a would-be comedian, who loves to look at the positive things about life. I saw life as partially a sitcom, but mostly a drama. I figured I could make it a fun-filled comedy.

When we were waiting in restaurants, I used to point out to Cyn my barometer of what I considered a relationship grown stale.

"See that couple over there. They said nothing to each other before eating, while eating, and afterwards. All of the things happening in the world, and they don't have a thing to say to each other. When our relationship hits that point, it will be time for me to move on."

What's really wonderful about being in a loving relationship is the chance to star or play a supporting role in so many mini-dramas, those emotional fluctuations aimed at affirming and perpetuating. Sometimes they're deep, shallow, up, or down, sometimes taking, and other times giving. They're love games, and they're played both consciously and unconsciously.

I always played games consciously. They were things I thought out and orchestrated. A man can't just leave something as important and difficult as trying to make a woman happy to chance.

And I wasn't being phony; I knew I was making myself a more interesting lover. Cyn was a natural, but she was too good to not have put a lot of thought into our relationship.

Love brings out a man's creativity, but sometimes we let it taper off, especially when a man assumes that he has his lover all locked up. Maybe because I wasn't married I considered myself a permanent suitor. I was in continuous pursuit of Cynthia, even though in the loving sense I believed I had her. She was my woman, my soulmate, and eventually my wife.

I think everyone will agree that the pursuit is the most exciting part of a union, so why not make an effort to keep laughing and living it up? This was a natural part of my persona, and Cyn fit right in as a complement and a challenge. She was genuinely funny and exciting, and I have a contrived silliness aimed at being entertaining.

If a woman did decide to leave me, I wanted her to be able to say that our time together was not stormy, and I wasn't about jealous fits and constant moodiness. I wanted her to analyze our stay together, and be able to admit that for the majority of time it had been good and that I had been a fun guy to be with. She didn't leave because of mistreatment, but because she was bored, or outgrew me.

I had a great peace of mind about women throughout all of the years I dated Cynthia. In spite of what some women might think, every man wants a strong woman who knows her own mind. No man wants to invest a lot of emotions into a woman who is weak-minded. Cyn was strong and I didn't fight her strength; I fed off of it. If a strong, good-looking woman wanted and loved me, it made me feel even better about myself.

Age, hard learning experiences, and lots of observation all helped me in bringing about that peace of mind. They all served me well in my long love affair with Cynthia, and I really believed that a man becomes a free man when he lifts the burden of trying to control women off of his shoulders. Aside from that, I thought I was hot stuff in the ghetto; I had a job and a car. I could easily be both of the most valued things career and professional women wanted: a chauffeur and an escort.

We men allow women to know us too well sometimes. We don't try to be mysterious like women do. We just say, "This is the way I am; accept it or leave it."

As the years passed, Cyn got to know my strengths and weaknesses too well. That was rather easy for her to do. She was secretive, but I'm a very open person. Like most women, Cyn felt as though she understood and really knew the real man underneath the macho facade and false image of a decisive decision-maker. She was cynical about men and their motives. When I would talk about how I was really into the equality of men and women, she said that the only equality that men really believed in was the equality of blame.

I used to always tell her, "You know Cyn, I really believe in the quote that behind every successful man there's a strong woman. Baby, never walk behind me; always be right here by my side."

The truth was, I really didn't like to place myself in the position where I only had myself to blame.

I believe in triumphantly beating on my chest, "I did it!" when something goes right, and saying "Baby... WE fucked up!" when something goes wrong.

That's one of the main perks in having a soulmate or a wife. Every man knows that women comes to a climax when they get a chance to scream at a man, "See! I told ya, you didn't know what the fuck you were doing!"

To avoid that, guys should let women in on the decision-making process, or at least let her think that she is.

Self-analysis is difficult. You're either going to make yourself look too good, too bad, or too foolish. As far as male chauvinism goes, I didn't mind being a "chauvinist of sorts." Chauvinism is a concept of gradation, and I think it's a part of masculinity until it becomes restricting or demeaning.

But I'm in no way a staunch male chauvinist. I think chauvinists are troubled, insecure men, he's right up there with racists, anti-Semites, homophobics, and fascists. I'm a humanitarian, and I believe in treating everybody fairly.

Cyn told me that I was a good man, and I'm going to take her word for it. She was past that stage of finding a no-good brother and trying to fundamentally change him.

Some women like to take on "projects," especially an exciting, handsome, or sexy guy. I know this type of man has a lot of women and my admiration. He has a reputation of messing over this woman and that woman, but to many women this makes him irresistible.

For some reason that escapes me; women believed they could change him, slow him down, and make him into somebody he's not. Some of these guys were extremely difficult projects, but some women still loved their dirty drawers. You know the type — a guy she took to see his first play, and he sat there with his hat on looking bored as hell, before he fell asleep during the second act.

Some women never learned that they can't change a man. Others, after going through the ritual of a few painful, failing "projects," are primed to except a different type brother.

Cyn tinkered with me, of course, but I did the same with her. You're going to always have to fine-tune a good relationship. I know she wouldn't have stayed with me so long, and she wouldn't have married me unless I was mostly a together brother, and of course, that's vice versa.

Something I Didn't Mean to Say

I just wanted to win an argument,
now I'm regretful... can't get it
    out my mind,

something I didn't mean to say.

I really didn't want to hurt her;
    maybe make her feel bad,
but I'm the one that's feeling bad,
    hurt, and it's all about

something I didn't mean to say.

    Thankfully
it's taught me a lesson about what
    love really is...

    love is
feeling each others' pain, feeling
pain received, feeling pain given,
    now I really
know the depth of my love for her,
    and it's all because of

something I didn't mean to say.

Enough

believe me brothers, I know,
 it's enough,
to have her at your side
to love her, cherish her
and build your life around her

if she loves you, she'll give
you more than enough of herself,

be happy with having her
and spend some time getting
to understand and know yourself

don't try to totally control,
understand, and possess her
... because you never will.

She Was Always Late

I was one of those impatient men
going out on a date or something,
sulking if she's late,
nearly blowing a splendid night
out on the town.

looking back, I wonder
how I could have acted that way?
she looked so pretty, and I was
so much in love,
"you're acting like a little boy,"
she would say.

it's common knowledge
that a woman's gonna be a little
late sometimes,
shoulda been more understanding,

nevertheless there was something
longing, prophetical,
loving in the silly way I acted,
in the missed minutes I couldn't
see and touch her, because today

adding them up,
seconds, minutes turn into hours,
hours into days and
that would've been much more joy,
precious togetherness,
I could have spent with my sweet,
sweet, sweet lover.

Domestication

There's nothing like the excitement of a new relationship with a woman that has stirred a feeling within you that you have not felt before. It was something that had started out as a trickle and quickly turned into a storm. There was always a sense of anticipation when I went to pick Cynthia up for a date. I would ring the bell and wait for her to come down from the third floor. Most of the times she was a little late, so I would wait in the car parked right in front of the building. It was a very short walk to the car, and my eyes stayed glued to the foyer to make sure she was safe. Sometimes I would wait by the door until she came down, because I wanted to touch her right away, get me some "sugah," and walk hugged-up to the car. But in the winter in Chicago, the "hawk" makes it no contest between chivalry and shivering, so I stayed in that car.

My eyes stayed glued to that foyer for another important reason; I wanted to see how good she looked that day or that night. She had this swift sexy swagger, a sassy version of the Chicago Stroll. The kind of walk women have when they know they look good. Along with her pretty smile and jazzy ambiance, that walk was the first assault on my senses. As she came closer, I was anxious to see how she had her hair. She had a basic style that she kept for a while, but she always added something a little bit different and alluring into it.

Cyn was a sharp dresser, and that was something else to look forward to. Was she slinky or high-fashioned? Did she have a soft look or look business-like? Lastly, I was also anticipating the fragrance she would be wearing, because she always smelled so good. My baby had all of that going for her with me; my anxiety was in just waiting to see her, but she didn't stop there. It seemed that in no time, she had become intuitive about my wants and needs. So she would occasionally bring down the finishing touch of the assault on my senses: a plate of home-cooked soul food in her hands. A woman walking out to my car with a plate of home-cooked food in her hands looked better than a super-model coming toward me on the runway. Arguably, a good home-cooked meal can make up for at least 10 defects in a woman. It means she's in touch with her primal and traditional role. This doesn't mean I believe a woman's place is in the kitchen. I have always dated working women, and I knew they didn't have any more time to spend standing over a stove than I did. I believed it was a sign that a woman really cared about a man. It told me that she was thinking about me when we weren't together; that I was on her mind while she was at work, sitting at her desk, and deciding what's for dinner. She was thinking about me while walking through the supermarket and when feeding her family. Nobody can tell me differently, I know how love works. There was care, thoughtfulness, and love in "dem dere collard greens."

The old wives' tale is true: "The way to a man's heart is through his stomach." And I am going to add that it is apparently the way to a woman's heart, too. The most successful pitch in getting a date in America is, "Would you like to go out to dinner?" Anyway, I remember saying to myself, "Damn Gamble, you've hit the jackpot. You've got yourself a pretty woman, and she can do more than just cook… she can burn."

Most bachelors believed rural southern girls were better cooks than urban women, they would cook more food when they cooked, and they didn't mind cooking for their man. These were generalizations, but there were some elements of truth in them. But it may not have been much of a sectional difference; I think it was a class and a feminist-type difference. I met women who would brag about not knowing how to cook, and they actually thought it was cute. I guess they were "Star-Trek" fans waiting for food replicators to be invented.

I really feel that a man isn't free until he can cook for himself. Thanks to frozen and canned food, I got to be an adequate cook. I don't believe that institutionalized lie that men make the best chefs. I want a woman to cook for me; it's something about a feminine touch. If a woman cares for you, her feelings are definitely fused into the taste, and that heightens its delectableness. The lie that men are better cooks was probably spread by men to keep women out of high-paying chef jobs. Men do all right, but they can't match a woman's touch. Next, we're going to hear transsexuals claiming that they're a better lay than a natural woman.

In those early days, Cynthia used that home-cooked meal hook to dig her claws deeper into me. It worked so well because I love to eat. Of course, I took her out to eat at a four-to-one ratio over her home cooking. This was fine with me; it was sort of the normal thing to do. Plus, I liked her introducing me to new restaurants. I had covered most of the South Side soul food restaurants, and Cynthia introduced me to a lot of Loop and North Side restaurants.

Speaking of cooking, there's one incident that happened a few years into our domestication years that I still think and laugh about. In our relationship there were the typical feminist vs. chauvinist predicaments, and there were predicaments coming from our ever-present country-boy vs. city-girl routines.

When I met Cynthia, I had been in Chicago for ten years. Being from Alabama, with a heavy Alabama dialect, gave me the opportunity to play the city-girl vs.

country-boy routine. It was all done in good-natured fun. Along with correcting my southern pronunciation of certain words, she used to get on my case for using older slang expressions. I recall her swearing that I used the phrase "I reckon" on our first date. She claimed she did all she could to keep from laughing out loud, but said she thought to herself, "Humm, I got me a big southern buck. All I have to do to confuse him is to ask him to conjugate the verb 'to be.' "

We had a lot of fun playing the city vs. rural routine. Of course, my view of our relationship was that I was southern bourgeoisie teaching a ghetto girl the social graces.

I guess it was inevitable for this routine of regional clashes to come to a head one day, and it did on one bright Saturday morning. I had taught her how to prepare a real breakfast for a southern man. This was different from the light-weight continental breakfasts you get at those Sunday morning brunches. She had learned that I didn't come to her house for breakfast or dinner to dine; I came to feed. Anyway, this breakfast included the works: porkchops, sausages, grits, eggs, hashbrowns, coffee, orange juice, milk, and some pancakes. She called and asked me to pick up some syrup on the way, and herein lies the crux of the problem. I called the incident "Syrupgate."

Everything was on the table when I arrived. Her mother, son, and daughter took their seats at the table when I walked into the apartment. Cyn was still in the kitchen bringing things out to the dining room. I was glad I caught her there, so I could tell her how good everything looked. She liked using her dining room for holidays when she would take out her pretty china and set a formal table. I liked that sort of thing, too, because at my place it was dinner mostly on paper plates. I was really glad to catch her alone, so I could get some morning sugah. This made the morning perfect, so far. Then I took out my favorite brand of syrup: Alaga. She said, "This is the best syrup you could get?"

"Yeah… that's the best there is. What's the problem?"

"We prefer Mrs. Butterworths to that Alabama/Georgia syrup."

"OK, next time I'll bring that watered-down stuff over here." That should have been the end of that for this morning, but she had strong taste preferences and name-brand loyalties that used to really get on my nerves. I sat down at the table with the others, and everyone dug in. She came in with her purse and announced that she would be back in a few minutes. She was going to the store to get some syrup. I said, "Wait, can't we just use this for today. Why go to the store now just to get some syrup."

Everybody had that awkward look on their faces. Her mother, forever the gracious lady, tried to smooth things over by asking her daughter to accept this for today and pick up some Mrs. Butterworths next week. Cyn decided to use the kids to bolster her viewpoint. They had sat there with that look on their faces that said, "Now you know how we feel when she gets in her mood."

Next, she actually opened the bottle, so they could get a whiff of the contents. And without them verbalizing an opinion, she had her boy go to the store and get some Mrs. Butterworths syrup. I just tore into the food with an added vigor. I pretended that nothing had happened. When it came time to eat the pancakes, I bathed them with Alaga, got a second helping, and ate like a maniac. I just sopped up the syrup until the plate was shining like it had been washed. She looked over at me wanting to laugh, because she knew I was mad as hell, but wouldn't say anything because her family was there. I was pissed and thinking to myself, "Lord, please do something about PMS."

I took my bottle of syrup home. That evening when I picked her up, we were on our way back to my place, and she had the nerve to ask me about it. She joked about it saying, "Baby, you're not still mad at me, are you? You know how particular I am. That's why I picked you over all of those men with money who were hitting on me."

I still didn't see anything funny about it,

"You want to show out in front of your family, huh? I'm going off the next time you're in one of your sapphire moods."

When the car stopped at the red light she reached over, pulled my head toward her, gave me a kiss on the jaw and said, "OK, my big buck... anything you say."

I think the woman was a little crazy. She just dismissed mood swings as though they never happened. But how could I stay mad at a crazy, sweet woman like that. I just shook my head and smiled it off.

My love affair with Cynthia was a long-running romantic comedy. Our story was a lot like some of my favorite situation comedies. There was a little of Ralph and Alice, and Cliff and Clair in our relationship. Those days were filled with laughter and a great deal of love. In my journal, I've tried to recreate some of that joy through scenes of common everyday occurrences in a regular relationship like ours. But my "chauvinist of sorts" views dominate, and consequently I end up looking like a chauvinist ranting against marriage and women.

Unfortunately, Cyn can't help me tell our story from her side, that strong, independent woman's side. Even though she was a butterfly feminist, she could give a stinging account of the injustices of marriage from a woman's side. And she could tear into male chauvinism with the best of feminists. At the time Cynthia came into my life, she was a woman that a man couldn't bullshit. She was just as responsible as I was for us not getting married for 16 years. I'm not sure what her answer would have been if I had asked her to marry me earlier on. I know she didn't see assuming the title of "a wife" as a panacea for her problems. In talking about her first marriage, she indicated that being a wife was restricting in many ways. She was happy with our relationship as it stood, and she had a "set place" for me in her life.

Cyn came from a job conference in New Jersey years ago, and told me that she was considering a transfer there, for more money and a higher level position. Now, I'm madly in love with this woman, and just like that, she was talking about taking a job in another state. I was cool outwardly. I calmly asked her for the details about how much money she was talking about, when, and whatever. But inside, I was screaming, "What about us?" I asked her, "You're not seriously thinking about taking that job, are you?"

She said, "Bobby, what would you do? Wouldn't you help your family out by making more money?"

I replied, "I guess I would."

She stayed overnight that evening, and other than her bombshell, we had a good night. But I couldn't sleep well at all. The thought of her leaving would awaken me every once in a while. I was shook up, sad, and pissed off. I started blaming myself for my predicament, "Gamble, this is what you get for having just one woman in your life."

That morning, she woke me up with a hug, saying sweetly, "Babe, you know I can't go that far away from you." Then she continued haughtily, "And you wanted to beg me to stay, didn't you? I thought you were gonna cry. I could see it on your face."

I was so damn happy, I didn't even respond verbally. I just held her tight and gave her a lot of wet kisses. Of course, I got arrogant as hell after I was convinced that she wasn't going anywhere. "Woman, I knew you couldn't leave me — even for a $100,000 more money."

Cyn played me like a drum that evening, and she never told me whether she was really considering an offer. It was an option that Cyn had as a professional, independent woman that I had never thought about until that night. And truthfully, my love and selfishness overrode my sense of fair play and equal rights.

I started thinking, "I'm gonna get me a welfare mother."

So you see, if Cyn could tell her side of our story, you would get a better picture of a strong woman playing the game like a man.

Our relationship spanned 18 years, and as it grew older, it became more and more like a marriage until we were finally married. I moved from being a boyfriend, to her man, to her soulmate, and eventually her husband. We met in 1975 and were married in 1992. I was a bachelor for a long time, and this status made me the object of admiration by most of my married male friends. Married men have the mistaken notion that a bachelor is totally free, or he pays just a little relationship dues. I knew it wasn't so. Still, there were things I used to fight against, because I believed they were domestication dues only married men should pay. There is one domestic chore that's at the top of the list. Although I loved home-cooked meals, I didn't like to go grocery shopping with Cyn, but I ended up doing it a lot. I didn't have to do this when I was just her boyfriend. It was when I became "her man" that going grocery shopping came into play. This was definitely paying heavy, time-consuming, domesticated, married man's dues. I preferred how a free bachelor operates.

A bachelor wisks through a supermarket in about 15 minutes. He picks up some beer, chips, and sweets to eat while watching the big game. I observed husband dues at its very worst in the supermarket. A line of men with sad hang dog looks on their faces, walking behind their wives slowly pushing a cart. The wife has a long check list in her hand, and a pleasant look on her face as though she's really enjoying herself. They're never satisfied with the cut of meat that's already out. This is a 20-minute stop alone while the butcher cuts and wraps new meat at her request. The canned soup section takes up 15 minutes. Would it be Campbell's or another brand? You would think she was making a major foreign policy decision. For every item, she stops and reads labels. Women routinely read labels as if they're checking for punctuation and subject/verb agreement. In the supermarket a wife is a mover and shaker. She's making decisions, directing the operation, checking off things, and occasionally turning and asking the husband what he might want. He's standing there nodding his head, following and pushing that cart like a teenager walking behind his mama. He may as well have his thumb in his mouth.

The husband's a bender and stacker. That's his main job besides paying for the groceries and reaching up and down on the shelves picking up the heavy articles. He has to make sure that various items won't be crushed, the items are arranged so that enough groceries that should be in two carts all get into one cart. It's sort of like him making bread and pork and beans corporate decisions. He has to put the items on the belt and wait for the teenager to put them in the shopping bags. Grocery bags fill up the trunk and the back seat of his car. He helped the teenager put them in the car, but the teenager won't be at his house to help him unpack. It takes five trips from the car to the kitchen. He's almost finished now, that is, after he helps put away the frozen goods. When he grabs a beer and flops down in his favorite chair, the game is at the two minute warning of the second half.

I've watched this comic scene replayed many times. I've said to myself, "Is this what a bachelor has to look forward to? I've been through this marriage scene before." I thought about the warrior tradition that makes up the multi-racial stock in America. The spirits of the Zulu, the Apache, the Viking, and the Samurai have retreated from the ferocity of the battlefield to walking meekly behind their wives pushing a shopping cart. I know there's more to marriage than that scene, and I concur that it can be a glorious institution, but domestication can also be funny as hell. That's why they make all of those sitcoms about it.

Cyn didn't drive a car, so I would take her where she wanted to go. At first I used to take her shopping for clothes. For some reason, this seemed to be less of a domestic stigma for a bachelor than grocery shopping, and I didn't mind it too much. Especially since she wasn't looking for a "sponsor," or a guy who was expected to pay for the clothes when he drove a woman shopping. Getting a sponsor, also called "sugar daddy," to buy them things goes back a long way in the relationship between a man and a woman. The modern woman, and the big city girl in particular, have refined this art. I was on the watch to see exactly what type of woman Cyn was during the first few times I drove her to the shopping centers. I guess I wasn't surprised to find that she wasn't the kind of woman looking for a man to buy her clothes. Later on, when the relationship became tight, that changed a little. She really liked my getting her accessories, and I liked to get them for her. She was such a sharp dresser that taking her to buy clothes was some heavy dues to pay in time if nothing else. There were times I thought I would never get out of "dem stores." I drove all over Chicago and Chicagoland. Except for the Loop, most of the other major shopping malls are located in the suburbs. Naturally this was a source of arguments sometimes. Maybe I was just being a typical male — very selfish and insensitive for placing my concerns about a major, slippery, street-clogging, dangerous, snowstorm on the way — over the possibilities of a woman missing a half-price sale.

I tried all types of pleasant rationales in an attempt to get out of taking her clothes shopping. I suggested that it was a girlfriends-type activity. She told me that girlfriends stayed out there too long and made too many unnecessary side stops. I was thinking, "And you don't. At least they want to be out there." Her clincher was always, "Baby, I want to be with you." And she had this way of grabbing my hand or placing her head on my shoulder when she said it.

At this time in our relationship, I had moved from being her boyfriend to her man, and that's a step up in some ways and a step down in others. Stepping down meant that my domestication dues were now similar to that of a husband. My lifestyle, the way I dressed, and the way I made love were all fair game for critiquing. Of course, she couldn't go as far as a woman with "papers." Those papers women talk about having on a man are like a license to abuse a man's free time. They also give a woman the go-ahead to work on his cure because most women see men as suffering from "high self-esteem."

The gradual erosion of freedom in a relationship with a woman starts from the high point during courtship, to boyfriend, her man, soulmate, and rock bottom, a husband. So just like a husband, I was now on twenty-four hour call. A man has to find a happy medium in paying dues just to keep from being surly all the time. After all, women have to pay some minute, but unpleasant dues too.

Although going shopping with a woman is mostly boring, there are some nice things about it. I was the type of guy that would be kicking and screaming when dragged from in front of the television, but when I got to where she wanted to take me, I enjoyed myself most of the times. I didn't like crowds, so I wouldn't attend the Taste of Chicago. But once she got me to go, I wouldn't miss it. I guess men are always complaining about women and shopping. I would always use this quote from a poet out of Atlanta called B-rap to get on Cyn's case about buying a lot of clothes. "A black woman will make enough money to run a household and she'll spend it covering her asshole."

Taking a woman shopping, and being with her while she's trying on dresses, is domestication similar to walking meekly behind her pushing the cart in the supermarket. A man's main job is to stand there like a zombie and hold her purse. There are hardly ever any seats around, so you can't get any reading done. I noticed that the men waiting on their wives or girlfriends didn't generally talk to each other. We glanced at each other, and there was a feeling of "brothers in bondage," but there was no "How's it going? What do you think about the Cubbies?"

It would be hypocritical to talk macho-talk here. After all, the macho men were at home. They were watching the game with their feet propped up and a beer in their hands.

Another reason the men were so quiet was because it was best not to say anything, especially about a woman's dress selection. I had found a seat this day. Cyn came out of the dressing room with this dress on, and she asked me how I liked it. I was just being honest saying, "It's OK. It looks nice."

A look of disappointment came over her face. She apparently loved the dress. She said, "Just OK?"

"Well, what do I know? You asked my opinion, and I gave it. If you really like it, buy it."

She took it off and brought it back for me to hold while she tried on another. She came back out and asked me about a fancier dress that I liked much better. I decided to be more vocal in my praise this time letting her know that I really agreed with her choice. "That's really sharp. Baby, that's you. Get it."

She looked at me funny, "You would like some gaudy, cheap stuff like this. I wouldn't wear this to a rummage sale."

I was taken aback. "You mean you went and tried on that dress to prove some kind of point?"

"Like most men, you don't know anything about women's fashion."

"I know what I like, and I know what most men like. You want to dress for your man, or you want to dress for the girls?" Anyway, it was a good lesson for me. I understood the zombies much better. A man can't win with a woman, so you sit there and say nothing. Thus the zombie-like expression, "I don't know nothing. Don't ask me nothing! Just hurry up."

A man fights domestication like hell because most women really have funny ways. It was a gimme that Cyn was going to be late, and I could accept that. Good things come to those who wait. But Cyn had this habit of not knowing when to leave. She had a lot of girlfriends, so there was always some social function she was invited to. I had to drop her off or go along. I would try to get her to stay home and rest when it was obvious she was bone-tired, but she was the type to say, "We have to at least make a short appearance."

My answer was, "Bullshit! People will understand if you just say you're out of it." A lot of times I went anyway. Other times I would drive her, and go home and wait for her call. Either way, it was when it was time to go that caused some problems. There's definitely a difference when a woman says she's ready to go and the actual act of leaving. When I was ready to leave, I would just get up and say, "I'm gone."

A lot of times a man is ready to go because his woman is looking good, he's had a few drinks, and he wants to hurry home and get her in the sack. Cyn was the type who insisted on staying a "respectable" amount of time. She couldn't just leave, she had to make a graceful exit. There was always chit-chatting at the door and prolonged good-byes. Many times I had to gently whisper in her ear, "Sweetheart, can we get the fuck outta here?"

"Bobby don't be so rude and ill-mannered."

I always believed I could have been more successful in my fight against avoiding the drudgery of paying so much in domesticated dues if I just could have taught Cynthia how to drive a car. I mean I really tried hard, and she tried hard, too, but it was just not to be. I know two men who were unable to drive a car after trying for a number of years, and a few women too, so I guess it's something some people, for whatever reason, can't learn to do.

Naturally, Cyn was unfazed by any quotes I came up with or any other teasing concerning her love of clothes. In reality, it was sort of hypocritical for me to criticize her in the first place. She was a dresser, and I loved the way she dressed. It was a part of her mystique, self-expression, creativity, and sensuality. A guy that says he doesn't like a sharply dressed woman is lying. It's just that when it's his woman dominating the closet space and running up credit card bills (even when she works) that his jaws get tight. But it's nothing for the same guy to compliment a woman at work.

I couldn't do much of anything to make going to the supermarket a more pleasant experience, but going to the Loop or to the mall was nice. It gave us a chance to try out several different restaurants. Fortunately for me, Cyn worked in the Loop. She could pick up things on her lunch hour or immediately after work. Her last Ameritech work station was located in the Apparel Center in the Holiday Inn. She could walk across the street to the shopping center in the Merchandise Mart without going outside.

Maybe lost in the shuffle of complaints about paying domestic dues is the fact that I was with the woman that I loved. We were doing this, doing that, holding hands, walking hugged-up, and even arguing sometimes. But looking back, these were technicolor days and technicolor times. I really miss them, just as I miss her. They'll always be a part of us together... sweet, precious, and unforgettable times.

Love on an Autumn Windy City Night

bluesy, dark
clear & chilly windy-city night,
autumn-air, breeze off the lake,
crescentic moonlight,

lovers love to cruise Chicago's
Lake Shore Drive
reptilian & tungsten-lit along
a bedarken lakeside,

Chicago's nighttime
electric skyline's colored like
a yuletide tree,

their first date is in the Loop;
they're on their golden jubilee,

bright city lights,
splendid dark night, strolling
in a hot, glorious love affair,
desirers
rapping "sweet-nothings" warms
the chilly Chicago air.

Flower Print Dress

It was loveliness and femininity
	accumulated...
	she and springtime
	Lake Michigan
	a lake breeze
	the look of love

and a long flower print dress.

	Hanging
loosely over her breasts,
clenching her small waist,
the dress was imprinted with
	colorful
flowers I couldn't recognize
	maybe
azaleas, geraniums, or daisies,

all on a bright saffron-yellow.

	It was made
of fabric I wasn't sure of,
	maybe
chiffon, rayon, silk, or cotton.

	When
it whiffed in the Lake breezes
it carried the scent of a sweet
	fruity cologne

	and
the gusty breezes pressed it
	against her body
framing her long slender thighs

It was a
beautiful technicolor evening,
sail boats
with multicolored sails moved
up and down on the Great Lake,

seagulls circled and screamed.

She's feline graceful
and moved very easily but kept
looking down as though she were
afraid
her Egyptian-looking sandals
couldn't safely
move over the large square rocks.

She worried
needlessly because I wouldn't
let anything happen to her,
I'm in love.

She's
addicting, tasty as ambrosia,
soft and delicate as rose petals

and she's
as pretty as the full blossoms
on her
saffron-yellow flower print dress.

When is a Woman the Happiest?

everyman
wants to know when a woman's the
happiest and moreso, when is her
happiness guaranteed?

when just being
in your presence, being near you,
touching you?

sometimes and sometimes not.

when driving along
with you in your fine shiny car?
mostly, especially when you're
running an
errand, chauffeuring, escorting.

when in your bed?
of course, if a man's skillful:
sets the mood, masters foreplay,
gives a vigorous performance,

she's happy
plenty a times but not everytime.

when she's "in a man's pocket?"

always!

ME AND HER: NIGHTS WHEN WE WERE HAPPY

Rivals on a Chicago Summer Night

Seductress night,
clear, starry, sweet-air night
filled with cool, cologned air,
glamorous one,
lean to my lips and I'll whisper
"dark girl I love you too."

Teasing night wind
swooping off the Cimmerian lake,
rustling trees,
slithering in my shirt caressing,
squinting my eyes,
sweetness ticklish on my tongue,
tasting of
vanilla, apples, jasmine, frappe,

because of you
I'm overflowing with love for her
my natural woman,
I'll knock on her door very soon
so I'll confess

the light in her eyes is brighter
than your stars,
her lips are warm and wetter than
your summer rain,
her touch is softer, her scent will
make your sweet air sweeter, but
sorceress night

don't be
chagrined, jealous, and possessive,
she outshines technicolor days too.

Wildflower

she's undeniably a flower,
pretty, scented, and fragile,
    sometimes
she looks like she'll break
at my touch, but she's more
a wildflower: a rugosa rose,
a wood lily, American Lotus,
independent, hardy, natural
she didn't need a man's
touch, care, and cultivation
    to bloom…

Like a lost honeybee I was
wandering when drawn to her

    she was
in full blossom, wide open,
prissy, moist, and inviting
I sensed that she was free
directed by her inner-self,

    intuitively
she sensed my fascination,
turned to me as if I were
the warm rays of the sun,
knowing I didn't want to
change her or control her

just love her and need her
    and drink of
her luscious, sweet Nectar.

Leaving the Lady Behind

She's my
first lady, educated, cultivated,
Delta Sigma Theta, sophisticated.
The lady
knows how to talk, has a swagger
in her walk, a devastating smile,

she wears the latest styles.

The lady
knows which way to vote,
the lady's poetical in her quotes,
she's under control, never gloats,

looks fantastic in a long fur coat.

The lady
prefers her gold in serpentine,
the lady's adaptable to any scene,
cooks down home or any cuisine,

the lady reads *Essence Magazine.*

The lady
orders a tall glass of white wine,
the lady's beautiful and feline,
the lady's graciousness sublime,
but when it comes to bedroom-time,

The woman
knows how to leave the lady behind.

The Hug

I really don't remember what the argument was about... well, maybe I do, but it's not important now. I distinctly remember being steaming mad. It was the feeling of being so pissed off that I didn't want to be in the same room with Cyn. I was going to finish listening to music and exile myself to sleeping on the sofa in the living room. Actually, if it came to that, I was going to sleep on the spare bed in the other room. That sofa wasn't comfortable enough for me to sleep on all night, mad or not mad.

Cyn finished whatever she was watching on television and came into the living room at the beginning of the news at ten. We hadn't been speaking, so I saw no reason to start up a conversation on something that we couldn't settle before. She just walked up and sat right beside me on the sofa. I started to say, "Woman, don't touch me," but I always thought that was a female way of acting during an argument. So I just lay there and said nothing. But she said, "Bobby, I know you're mad, but I'm not going to talk about it anymore. I'm not going to apologize. I don't have anything to apologize for. But you should apologize. Meanwhile, I'm going to lie right here, and I'm going to hug you until you stop acting like a ten-year-old, spoiled little boy." And she was pushy as hell, just telling me, "Move over!"

I had already removed the three big pillows from the sofa. I was using two of them as head pillows. Then she worked her right arm between that space where the big pillows I was resting on prevented my back from being flat on the sofa. She pulled my left arm over her shoulder, placed her head on my chest, and her left arm across my body. I had taken those pillows off the sofa to give me more room, and I was lying in the center of the sofa before her body had pushed me back.

She didn't say anything else, but hugged me as she said she would. Even though my arm was across her shoulder, I kept as little pressure on it as possible. I wasn't about to squeeze her back, and I had started scheming. I was thinking about lying there for a while just to show her that this touching and hugging wasn't having any effect on me. Then without saying anything, I was going to remove her arm, get off the sofa, and go to my other room to sleep for the night.

I guess that wasn't a really bad thing to do. Arguments are common in relationships, and many escalate into various things that are much worse than simply sleeping in separate bedrooms. But it was a big event for us because we expected the same things out of our relationship. We were not married, living together, paying bills, or rearing children together. We were soulmates and lovers on a long, unofficial honeymoon. We expected the times we were together to be no less than pleasant. If other lovers wanted to have a stormy love affair, more power to them. Neither Cyn nor I was going to remain in a bad relationship — a relationship where there were frequent arguments, ruined nights, and frequent breaking up and getting back together. Every argument that ended up ruining a pleasant night, a night when we were not a comfort to each other, just didn't sit well with either of us.

I didn't go to the other room because that hugging had begun to work on my anger. It was helped out a little by the scent of her hair and her softness, but mostly it was just the act of her hugging me. She said she wasn't going to apologize, but I had taken it as an apology, if not an outright capitulation. I know I had tried to save a night by apologizing and hugging, and had been met with the female "Don't touch me" attitude on many occasions.

Soon Cyn asked me if we were going to sleep on the sofa for the rest of the night. I said, "You don't have to."

She said, "I want to sleep with you. You know that."

It took me about thirty seconds to answer, "I can't move."

Lying there, it occurred to me that anger was like a third person in the room. Somebody there who would not allow us to do what we both really wanted to do, which was to be sweet and loving when we were together. But things had started working just like she had expected them to do. The anger was draining out of me as she held on to me. It started at the top of my head and drained right down through my guts. Every few minutes gave me more peace of mind. Earlier she had looked up at me a couple of times, trying to make eye contact, but I had kept staring straight ahead. You play so many games when you're angry it becomes instinctive, and you're a little out of control. Still, a new understanding of things happened that night. I realized that together we could gang up on anger. We could beat that invisible third person in the room that kept us from being sweet to each other. But anger is like a hot stove, you just have to wait for it to cool off. I wanted to but couldn't put my newfound logic to work right away. I was thinking, "What is this really? Is this the tender trap, and had I fallen right into it? What about all of those times when I had tried to make up, and she said, 'Don't touch me.'"

Anger wasn't going to let me rationalize my way out of this situation easily; after all, it's an emotional creature. But I said to myself, "Since men are logical, I should naturally take the lead in this situation." I felt stupid as hell about not being grateful that she didn't escalate matters. She was trying to save the night from separate beds. I was feeling a little foolish, even guilty, and debating with myself as to whether I should hug her back and say, "OK babe, let's get up and go to the bedroom."

The debating with myself ended abruptly when I heard her snore-like breathing. I was thinking, "Wait a minute; ain't this a bitch. This woman fell asleep on my argument. I'm uncomfortable as hell on this damn sofa, and she's sleeping peacefully. I'm the one who should be asleep. She should be awake, hugging me and trying to get me in a better mood. How can a woman just go to sleep while her man is in mental pain? Obviously, she wants to wear the pants in this relationship. Next she's going to want to start pissing standing up."

Instinctively I was still playing that war of the sexes game. Even as much as I wanted to get up and sleep in my soft comfortable bed. I decided to macho my way to the bedroom without her thinking that she had soothed the savage beast, and that he, with his head down and balls deflated, was going meekly to the bedroom. Instead of hugging her like I really wanted to, I came on hard. "Hey! Wake up! You're hurting my neck. Let's go get in the bed."

Softly, sweet, and apologetic, she said, "Oh, I'm sorry baby." And as we were getting up, I just grunted something back. While we headed for the bedroom, I was thinking, "Ugh, such a sweet, precious thang. I really wish I could be sweet to her all the time, but she can piss me off for no reason sometimes."

The argument was about what used to be called the old headache excuse. I think men have a stronger sex drive than women, and we are insensitive sometimes in our approach to them. Because we can perform sexually, anytime and anywhere, we forget that women are different. Women are more romantic, and they have to be in a certain mood. But at the same time, I think women should also be more sensitive to what the man is going through. Our strong sexual drive is based on the survival of our species, and we are in a natural state of anxiety and aggressiveness in an attempt to satisfy that drive.

Anyway, the old headache excuse is hardly used by

women anymore because it isn't necessary. As soon as women became more of a political and economic force in America, they acted like Pharaoh and had the word "obey" stricken from the marriage vows. I don't recall the year or even the decade, but I remember that it was once a part of the bride's promise. In the "good ole days" men had the force of law and custom on their side. Now we're beggars, bribers, and pouters. That's why I ended up like a fool, a six-foot-three man lying on a five-foot-ten sofa. And my legs were cramped, back hurting, neck hurting, had a hard-on, and my mouth was stuck-out pouting.

That hug really defeated Mr. Anger. When we got in bed, I hugged her, got me some sugah, and said, "You know Cyn, that was real nice of you to help me out of that bad mood. You know me… anger comes slow to me, but it leaves even slower. It helps when you aggressively help me chase a bad mood away. We should always use a good hug until our anger subsides."

"Bob, I don't know if I can bring myself to do it all the time."

"If you don't mind me saying it, it's mostly the woman that cries 'don't touch me.'"

Then I just outright said, "Cyn I need that. I can't stop myself from playing games, and you can't either sometimes. All it takes is getting rid of the ego or the feeling that one of us is giving in." Hugging became one of our staples in an argument because it works. So my advice to other couples is, if you're mad and you feel that you can't make up right away, and you absolutely don't want to be touched, try to do it anyway. Time together is too precious to throw away. I don't know whether hugging was impromptu on her part, or if she had read about it somewhere. There are books and articles about hugging and making up. Still, it's not easy to do when you're pissed-off. But on that night, I meant it a little bit more when I said, "Good night, babe, you're all right, I love you."

Body Scribble

Saturday morning
in the first, faint light of dawn
I was awakened by a soft scribble,
with her eyeliner
she had scribbled her name with
an apostrophe "S" above my navel
I grabbed the eyeliner before
she placed it on the night stand,

she looked so pretty,
even without makeup on her face,
a natural beauty, a natural woman,
her partially covered hips curved
sharply,
staring and breathing heavily her
bellybutton rising up and down,

I scribbled my name
with an apostrophe S on her belly;
we said nothing to each other,
just turned and went back to sleep.

Showering together,
the words faded from our flesh but
I don't believe they disappeared
in swift, soapy-water,

those words saying
"we belong to each other" raced
through our blood streams right
into our hearts,
a place where they will always be.

Painting on a Canvas of Flesh

she would paint in the mirror
  right before
heading for work or going out
just unpretentiously coloring,
  glossing her lips,
something routine, but surely
sheer manipulative femininity
  for a man
and she probably never thought
  about my impression,

  vulvate erogenous
I couldn't stop from watching
  glossy, parted lips
I would stare at them while
  she was sleeping,

  they're chiseled
fleshy, nubian, expressive
the V indentation's slightly
off-centered and swept-up
  on one side,

think about them all the time
moist, soft, cinnamon-sweet
  want them
smiling, staring back at me
whispering and exhaling heat
  hoping she'll
forget smearing, fading gloss
  I need them on me.

The Terry Cloth Robe

Most of her makeup had faded, her face was a little shiny, and her hair had that disheveled look like she had pulled a tight sweater off over her head. Cyn had on this thick, blue terry cloth robe. The kind advertised as "one size fits all." Tonight, she had an earthy sex appeal. The kind those pretty, dancing, sweating, female aerobic instructors have, but her arms looked too weak to forcibly serve a tennis ball. They looked like they were made for squeezing or throwing kisses.

One of her legs was dangling off the side of the bed. The other was drawn up leaning slightly across her body. She was painting her toenails red with her right hand, and she was balancing herself with her left. As I watched her, I was thinking about a scene in the movie *Carmen Jones*. We had watched it recently on television, and I had fallen in love with Dorothy Dandridge when the movie first came out. There was this great scene where Dorothy Dandridge asked Harry Belafonte to blow on her toenails to dry them. I was thinking that the scene was in the summer time, so I asked Cyn, "Why are you painting your toenails when you're no longer wearing your feet bare in sandals?"

She sort of waved her feet saying, "Don't you think that's pretty? Don't you like them?

"Sure, yeah."

"Do I need more reasons than that?"

"I guess not… Can I watch?"

"Un-huh."

In a few seconds she said, "Come here and paint my left foot; my arms and back are tired. Can you do that without messing up?"

"Sure babe. Next you want to play Dorothy Dandridge in *Carmen Jones* and ask me to blow them dry, right?"

"Yeah, if you were Harry Belafonte."

I came back fast, "And if you were Dorothy Dandridge I would beg you to let me suck on them."

"I knew you had some freak in you; just don't paint my skin."

I took my time and was doing a pretty good job, but I wasn't prepared for the intensified loving feelings and the sheer eroticism of the scene.

"One down, four to go. You know Cyn, as nervous as I am, I'm surprised I was able to do that so well."

"Bob, it's just painting nails. You're not doing brain surgery."

"It's brushing against your baby softness. Just being this close to a pretty lady has always made me stumble and bumble. You know... like a first-grader trying to show off in front of his girlfriend. Cyn, I don't think I'll be able to finish this."

She pulled my head and kissed me on the cheek, "Baby, you sho' know how to lie good sometimes, but keep painting, you've been hired."

Talk about magic moments, this was it. I was sitting next to her on her left side, and she was leaning back on both hands. My right arm was across her left leg which was bent at the knee. I held her feet in my left hand right up over my lap. I could smell her cologne. Blending with her natural scent, it was so magnetically pheromonal.

When I had finished with her nails, she told me I did a good job and that she would allow me to paint both feet next time.

It was an impromptu request on her part in asking me to do her nails. She was tired, not being flirtatious, and she didn't seem to be aware of its sensual overtones. Even for me, it was an unexpected pleasure. So I held on to that closeness, brushing against her softness, and savoring the pheromonal scent of Alyssa Ashley's musk cologne.

I think there are very few moments when a woman looks sexier than those times when she has on a bathrobe. I'm talking about the robe itself, and what it does for the female physique and the feminine mystique. It doesn't matter about the size of her frame. She could be petite or large, but nature is uniform in making her waist smaller than her hips, and a tightly-pulled belt on a robe brings this out like nothing else that she wears. For Nubian beauties, accurately described by Sir Mix-A-Lot as having nice "back," this is accentuated sexuality.

My favorite type of robe on a woman is a terry cloth robe. Silk or satin is tied for second. Cyn looked good in either type. She had a full bust and a slender waist. Silk and satin are long, clinging, and expertly show off the female figure. But a terry cloth robe seems to have been made for warmth. It's fluffy and oversized, as though by design, it's made for tantalizing by concealment of that "assortment of goodies." Therein lies all of the fun; the unraveling of fabric and of passion.

That night she had on my terry cloth robe, the kind with a hood on it. And it looked much better on her than it did on me. Anyway, I was trying to hold on to that spontaneous, magic moment. Everything seemed to have been in place. When I looked in her eyes, she stared back at me with that "Well, boy" look; as in, "Well boy, what are you gonna do?"

After years of going out together, I had virtually discarded one of the cardinal rules of bachelorhood: never allow a woman to answer your telephone. But there was really no reason she shouldn't answer my phone. For a long time, there was just she and I. She knew this, but sometimes a girlfriend can't resist the thrill that one day she will answer her man's phone, and a sweet talking rival will be on the other end.

The phone rang, Cyn answered it, and it was for her. The call wasn't from her daughter, mother, nor was it an important message from her job. Neither was it an annoying insurance salesman, nor the Red Cross with orders to evacuate the city. It was the worst of all people to be calling at a time like this, a close girlfriend with problems. A safe bet would be that it was man problems. Some woman who loves some guy more than she loves herself. Instead of getting him out of her life, she was calling... again... to cry about something he had done, or something he didn't do. Just saying to myself a barely audible but heartfelt "Agh, shit!" helped me out a little.

However, for the skillful suitor this situation can be turned around sometimes. You can be free to maneuver and force your lover to hang up, even on a girlfriend. First, I paused for a while to cool off my mood. Also, so Cyn could exercise common sense and get that girlfriend off of the line by herself. But I looked at her face when she said a long and loud, "Whaat?" I knew then that this was the beginning of a long, girlfriend gripe session, a talk-a-thon. That long "what" was followed by removing her leg from my lap and fully covering up with the robe. She turned on her side away from me, and she got in a comfortable position with that telephone glued on her ear.

Even still, I was not about to just give up on that magic moment and go watch television. The "master" was plotting his moves. A woman is in a vulnerable position to moves when she's on the telephone. But this was not to be; Cyn was definitely going to listen sympathetically to a girlfriend. I planned on waiting some respectful minutes before I was ready to let her read my lips and get that girlfriend off MY telephone line.

A lot of Cyn's girlfriends had my phone number, and

she received calls at my place on a regular basis. If any friends called her apartment and she was at my place, they were given my number to reach her. She called out a lot too. Many evenings we just seemed to be under the same roof instead of on a date because she used the telephone until she hit the sack. I was comfortable with her using my telephone because she was over a lot, and I considered my place as our place. Both of us had some job-related work to do on many occasions. We were not constantly relating to each other; we just shared the same space sometimes. Besides work-related activities, I was more into TV drama shows, and she was more into comedies. So a lot of times I would be in another room watching my shows. Cyn liked sports, but not enough to sit and watch a game on TV.

Tonight I had planned to stay in the room with her so I wouldn't lose that physical connection. I didn't want to show any negative vibes just because the telephone rang at the wrong time. I made this gesture to her to indicate that I understood that we had been interrupted, and I knew that she was just as disappointed as I was. I moved to her other side where she could see me and turned the television down. I put a pillow under my neck, and lay down half-way on the bed with my feet on the floor. I draped my left arm across her legs and scooted close to make sure we were touching. The old "rub the body move" worked from this position sometimes.

In a few minutes when I felt the time was right, I sat up and gently squeezed her calf. Looking at her intently, I blew a kiss and mouthed, "Get her off the phone."

She looked back at me and kept talking without saying anything. I let a few more minutes pass before turning to her again. This time I pulled her robe back, kissed bare flesh, and mouthed a little more emphatically, "Get her off the phone!"

She told her girlfriend, "Wait a minute," then put her hands over the telephone, pulled that robe back closed, and told me, "This is important!"

I was thinking, "What! Tell that bitch to call a psychiatrist. Do they think I'm running a fucking lonely hearts clinic?"

It didn't look like the homeboy was faring too well, but this was a time for patience; the magic moments could still be saved. But soon there was an ominous sign that I knew would make everything more difficult. She had repositioned herself into a more comfortable position, and she had gotten into the dreaded "um-um-um" mode of listening.

Cyn was a great telephone talker and listener. She could go for long minutes without saying a word. Most of the time she would get into this rhythmical "um-um-um" response. It wasn't a straight monotone because she would occasionally change to a higher pitch on the first "um." Sort of like "UM-um-um." The ums were separated every few minutes by a "Girl, no!" or "He didn't." I knew that the girlfriend was talking about how some guy had done her wrong, and how sorry the brothers were in general. I was sitting right there when Cyn looked straight at me and said, "Girl, none of them are any good."

All I tried to do was to be romantic with my woman, and before I knew it I had become a victimizer.

I was getting really pissed because before I knew it these two women had me mad at a poor, innocent brother. Until I caught myself, they had me thinking that some guy I didn't even know was royally fucking up my night. But I started thinking correctly, and I planned to just persevere on my original mission. I turned on the low-light lamp, turned off the television, and I left the room. I turned on some soft music that she could hear in the living room, and proceeded to fix both of us a drink. I made myself a Jack and ginger and I took her some white wine.

I came in the room, sat on the side of the bed, and motioned her to stop for a minute. She told her girlfriend to wait a minute and placed her hand over the phone. It was one of my line's time. I concede that most of my lines were corny as hell, and they were meant to be humorous. But the effectiveness of any line is in its timing, the overall mood, and its sincerity. Plus, Cyn liked my lines, either corny or hitting the spot, and that was good enough for me to keep on keeping on.

"Hey, pretty lady, here's your favorite drink. Don't mind me being lonely, neglected, sitting in the living room all by myself. Talk as long as you need to. You know I'll take you anyway I can have you. Another thing Sweetheart, I want you to always refer to me as, 'Your toy,' and I'll always refer to you as, 'My joy.'" Then I grabbed her hand and kissed it before placing the long-stemmed wine glass in it.

Here came that pretty smile. Her reaction was that type of smile which is really more like a smirk, but it told me that she was thinking, "This boy is really trying hard."

So she gave me a wink and smacked a kiss before her first sip. I knew then that all I had to do was to go and relax to the music, enjoy my Jack Daniels, and wait for her to call.

She had one sip of wine left when she hung up the phone in a little less than 15 minutes. Her voice was sweet, like babytalk, when she called to me in the living room.

Wanting

I want her softness on me
I want her flavor on me
I want her breathing on me
I want her sweating on me
she has her spell on me.

Sequence

Sure, babe!
Like clockwork.
I'm a grandmaster
at unfastening.

What the?
Okay … maybe not
smoothly sometimes.

I'd love to…
Ugh!
they're very pretty;
can you make an arch?

Where?
If you want me to

Un-huh…
good and all night

And I really
really love you too.

Wetness

when it's wet, it's more than being
liquidy, juicy, searing, pheromonal

when it's wet, it's much more than
loveliness, open, rosy, quivering,
  wetness releases, transforms

in the sweet moments... in the dark
strained, guarded inhibitions are
    unlearned, surrendered.

    urbaneness, elegance
revert into the rhythm, noisiness
and naturalness of the rain forest,
and it's hotter, sloshy, sonorous

    and biting
in the sweet moments... in the dark.

Animal Syntax

honeyed-voice, solicitous
    exhorting,
nuances rising and weakening

    animal syntax,
although subtle and polished

    sometimes
in a sweet, primly urging,
    sometimes
a repetitiveness guttural
    and vulgar

I'm wrapped in woman's-meat,
    silky, fragrant,
hot, thrusting and slippery

couldn't help but obey her,
hold on, ride on, because

    her purring,
heated and blowing in my ear,
repeated "harder!" repeated
    "deeper!"

Afterglow

eyes closed, exhausted,
    can't move
breathless … tingling,

love and happiness
are raging brushfires
protracted, lingering,
    running
through our bodies

and we are simmering.

I'll hold on to her,
feeling her, smelling her,
until early morning because

    when a man
really, really loves a woman
the afterglow is never over.

Morning: Woman in My Soul

She's gone,
from the room, the house,
but as always
she's still wherever I am,
the woman is in my soul.

The earrings
she didn't choose sparkled
in formation on my dresser,
the powder-blue
embroidered silk slip she
wore yesterday gracefully
draped over a bedroom chair.

The air
was scented with her flavor,
instinctively I reached and
pressed her slip to my face,
breathing in
its closeness, its silkiness
and femininity.

I'm in love,
I wiped scented powder from
my face and the print of my
wet lips on silk dried fast.

In that primeval dawn light
just had to savor her again,
feel something of her again;
she's
ambrosial, moving through
my life spreading love and joy,
the woman is in my soul.

MELODIES FROM A WIND CHORUS IN JANUARY

Eschikagou

When in those places where
somebody needs somebody
and love flourishes,
we all huddle bracing
for the lightlessness days,

        straddling the
center of that land frozen
        in glacier times,

        it left an
inland sea while retreating
        blue, wide, deep,
great-waters the Chippewa
        called "mici gama,"

        and it left
a place of plains, marshes,
wild onion fields, savannas,
woodlands the Potawatomi
        called "Eschikagou."

        In
pre-Columbian times when
the Gods of the wind ruled

bitter winter nights

east winds from across the
deep, great waters wailed
        orchestral,

and the wind harmonized with
    the love chants
of Sacs, Foxs, Potawatomi,
for as smoke spiraled from
rows of buffalo-hide lodges,
warm flesh pressing together

panted and moaned in crescendo.

    In our time
winter's still hard in Chicago,
    but a windy city winter
has an austere, fierce beauty
that's very special for lovers.

When the winds howl and race
    unimpeded
off a frozen Lake Michigan,
wailing and snaking through
    Loop canyons of
ice-laden skyscrapers, the
black night is bitterly cold,

you don't want to sleep alone.

Crystals, squalls, drifts,
    splendid,
though tenaciously wintery,
nurture the desire to be
    together,

loving and warm and touching
and laughing and whispering

and snuggling
while the wind chorus sing
on the windowsill and
flurries are soft-painting

visions of Christmas scenes
etched deep in our memories
in pretty glossy-red
holly-green and silver-tinsel.

As the
black night grows older,
pompous winds are violent
dangerous ... but lyrical
roaring, then whispering
bellowing, then murmuring
giant trees bow in homage
but I have no fear of the
Wind God Aeolus,
rattling the wrought iron
of unyielding storm doors.

Though its awe and beauty's
overwhelming,
it comes this way too many
times for apprehensiveness.

Our houses are
stronger than buffalo-hides,
warmer than great campfires,
the storm has
become aphrodisiacal and the
wind chorus is singing
love songs on my windowsill.

By the Light of the Snow

The sun was dragging a darkness across the sky, but the darkness, not wanting to follow, was resisting. It was a tug-of-war, and it created a momentary stalemate because the sun was stranded on the edge of the horizon longer than usual. After a while, the sun disappeared, and it just as well, because it had done nothing to help warm the biting winter air.

It was dark, but even with the sun gone the freezing, silent night was not in total darkness. The ground was covered with pure-white snow, and it had turned on its reflecting lantern. It was a soft, diffused, natural glow, an illumination that's unlike any other.

The snow had covered roof tops — only the forms of cars could be seen, and limbs of tall trees looked skeletal lining the deserted streets. The scene was clean and beautiful.

Cyn and I trudged along on deep tire grooves right in the middle of the street. We occasionally moved aside to let the cars brave enough to venture down the side streets roll slowly by. Even though it was a full three weeks after Christmas, there were still colorful Christmas lights in windows, and there were lights blinking on evergreen shrubs in the front yards of the rows of bungalows.

Since it hadn't been a white Christmas, it was great to see Christmas lights still shining in some windows. They added an authenticity to the beautiful Christmas-card like scene. Sentimental Christmas carols were playing in my head, but otherwise the only other sounds were our heavy panting from trudging, and the crunching sound of old snow under a fresh covering of snow.

Though it was freezing, our love was very hot for each other. Happiness blanketed us like the beautiful snow covered the ground. I stopped and pulled the scarf down from around her mouth. Her breath was frosty steam, and I followed the steam to her cold lips, to her warm, wet tongue. After a sweet kiss, I started talking in my normal arrogant manner.

"Hey babe, you'll walk five miles in the snow just to get in my bed, huh?"

Jivey as always, she said, "I'll walk ten."

After a couple of kisses, our faces warmed just a little, and I responded, "Ten miles, huh? All right pretty lady, I'll believe anything you tell me."

As we kept panting and trudging, she said, "Baby it gets real warm in a fur coat."

"I know Cindy. That's why I bought you one."

"What! You didn't pay a penny, not one cent on this coat!"

"Woman, I'm taking care of the entertainment expenses of this relationship, and that allows your budget to free up the expense for a fur coat."

"Yeah, right."

I was able to say "Listen carefully"... before she stopped me.

"Here we go again. You're about to repeat the brother's favorite promissory note."

Then she mimicked a guy's voice, "Baby one day I'm going to buy you this, or buy you that... When I get the money."

"Woman, the brother was right. Cyn, you women need to make up your minds. Do you want to be kept, controlled, and jump when we say jump, or you wanna be independent and finance your own conspicuous consumption?"

Just like that, it went on and on as we trudged along heading for my place. Nothing unusual happened. We said nothing or did anything profound. But love isn't fueled by the unordinary. It needs no faraway, sunny place.

We were in the coldest month, on a freezing, snow-filled night in the windy city. It wasn't a South Pacific Island, but I felt like we were in paradise.

The power of love is fueled by togetherness, anyplace and anytime. Love makes the ordinary exciting and unforgettable.

So after every heavy snowfall in the middle of January, it becomes more than another winter night. When Christmas lights are still shining in some windows. When snow covers the ground and roofs of bungalows. When only the forms of cars can be seen, and limbs of tall trees lining deserted streets look skeletal.

I'll always think of her on that dark night when the snow turned on its lantern, that January night long ago. Maybe with a little sadness, but mostly with joy.

If I've learned anything about life, it's that there are a few things in life that last forever, and love and memories are two of them.

Sing Softly

wind-chorus on my windowsill
play our song just right,

make it sweet, loving too,
and sing it through the night.

Eschikagou Winter

SNOW STORM

The snow was melting and dripping off her tall leather boots; her fur coat lay sprawled across my sofa. It was one of those Friday nights after a hard work week. I didn't want to fall asleep, and I didn't want to stay awake. We danced slowly on the livingroom carpet, to "Patti" and she drank white wine from a long-stemmed glass, which bore her print of cherry lipstick around its rim.

It was divine isolation, cabin-fever style. It was an aloneness felt only in those loving times before a family was born, or after a family had moved away. She rose on stockinged feet, pulling the back of my neck to meet her moist, sculptured lips. She sprinkled a few kisses and whispered, "Baby, I'm bone-tired."

I was too, but I whispered back something silly, "You can't hang with me, huh?"

Our jobs were really the victimizers on most Friday nights. They halted stepping out and love games sometimes, but not inseparableness. Luckily, she wore no hair rollers on Fridays. That was a sure sign of when a girlfriend is used to you. It was too early for me to have even thought about going to bed, but it was obvious she was sleepy and planned on hitting the sack. Now I was free too, so to pass the time, I brought out a video tape of one of the season's Bulls victories.

When I reflect on that night, it has become a part of the feelings I have about my future. My future seems to be uncertain, and it's also on hold. I feel as though all of the good times to come for me in my future are in my past. So I keep replaying special nights in my head, over and over, as though they were some of my favorite black-and-white movies.

Still, that night was just one of the many special times in our love affair — a time when intense, elevated, loving feelings came over me without warning. But it was not always in a private place where warm bodies are touching each other. Sometimes it was in the Loop. Sometimes it was being together at a formal affair, while circulating around the room not knowing where she was at the moment. But I knew that she was there somewhere, and when it was time to leave, she would be leaving with me.

The feelings that had come over me pushed me up to a level I couldn't have reached alone. They were a part of a fusion that came from two people, and this merging of strong, loving feelings isn't rare. It's universal and primordial. It connects us with lovers of many different cultures, a connection over the expanse of time. A great part of this love involves protective feelings. Probably it is the same feeling felt by an Amazulu male embracing his bride while they overlook the wide banks of the White Umfolosi River, basking in the beauty of the green, rolling hills of Zululand. It's a close feeling of love, like the loving feelings of Mayan lovers on the top of a pyramid in Tikal, staring at the sky on a dark, billion-stars night.

During the height of being in love, at this zenith when all seems to be right with the world, there was a foreboding feeling that crept into my consciousness every once in a while. I allowed my mind to race ahead and feel the fear that most of us who are deeply in love have experienced on some occasions. It was the fear that my perfectly satisfying relationship with my irreplaceable lover would one day end too soon. It would not necessarily have been because of somebody else, but because of something dreadful and unknown. I didn't want to feel this way. No lover does, but fearful and negative thoughts can just creep into my mind. They crashed my beautiful, glorious party like a joyless interloper. But mercifully, the doubts and fears came in brief, fleeting melancholic moments, and didn't consume my being. It was as if sadness wanted to share the stage with joy for a flash cameo and then disappeared. I learned to look at those feelings as part of the price of love. I just moved on and enjoyed all of the blessings that were showering down on us.

Before starting the video tape of the game in my living room, I helped tuck Cyn into bed ever so gingerly. It was with a carefulness I had learned when I was a father to my two-month old son. After all, she was my baby now, and Cyn used Johnsons' Baby Lotion to help soften her skin which was already baby soft. Cindy must have been really tired because her eyes were closed as soon as her head hit the pillow. I pulled the covers over her shoulders and sat on the side of the bed, touching her hair. I was trying to get me some goodnight sugah, but ended up alternating kisses on her eyebrow and jaw. I couldn't kiss her on the lips, because she was moving her head around trying to get me to leave her alone, but I was pushy and persistent.

"Sweet thang, can I get some real goodnight sugah?" I asked sweetly.

She didn't open her eyes, but turned her head from the pillow toward me. In a wispy, half-sleep voice she murmured, "Goodnight, Babe."

She tried to give me a quick smack on the lips, but I took what I wanted, a long kiss right on the mouth, while we breathed and fought for the same air.

Briefly satisfied, I broke off so I could get me some sweet neck-sugah. She didn't resist this move because it allowed her to press her head back into her pillow. I paused on the neck for a while, sniffing in the sensual blend of her natural scent with her perfume. I closed my eyes and drew in her essence, that willowy femininity she overflowed with. "Me and you," I whispered for the umteenth time. It was one of my favorite expressions for letting her know how deeply I loved her. She responded with a sleepy, "I love you, too. When are you coming to bed?"

"When I finish the game."

Her eyes finally popped open, "The game! Tonight? You, must be sick."

She closed her eyes and turned back into the pillow, "Baby, come to bed with me."

"For what, you're asleep already."

"No I'm not. You know I can't sleep without you."

"Yeah, right. Looks like you're doing OK to me."

"Bobby, are you coming?"

"First… say you can't live or sleep without me."

"I can't live or sleep without you."

"All right, but you know it's not even eight-thirty yet."

"Just come and hold me until I go to sleep."

I used to lie with her while she went to sleep many, many times. Then I would carefully slide out of the bed and do whatever I had to do. She worked really hard, and she still had to come home and do things for her family. She was just plain tired a lot of times. My place was a refuge where she didn't have to do anything but look pretty, rest, and be waited on.

When she had asked me to lie with her that night until she went to sleep, I must have paused or something. She was annoyed and snapped at me with a sharp, "Goodnight, Bobby."

I know she would have been asleep if I hadn't bothered her for some sugah. I should have readily jumped under the covers with her, but this would have meant that I would have to undress. I had planned on getting a shovel and knocking the snow off of my steps that night while it was fresh and light. Anyway, first things first.

The sheets were cold, except where she was lying. When she felt me snuggling up behind her, she arched her back closer to me, but didn't turn over or open her eyes. She just reached her arm back and touched me on the face. I grabbed her hand and kissed it in the palm. I was determined not to keep her from going into a deep sleep, so I just whispered things quietly enough for only me to hear. You know… just being braggadocio as men are sometimes.

"I don't like the way you said goodnight. It wasn't sweet enough. Woman, you're with a man that's in demand. Do you have any idea how many fine women would like to be right here where you are? Here in my bed."

She didn't hear me, or she just didn't answer. I was on my side with my elbow propped and leaning with my jaw in my hand. I was a happy man, deeply in love with a woman who loved me. This was another night when I felt that life had been really good to me. I planted a kiss on her bare shoulder blade, and whispered, "OK girl, I know you've got me, but don't get too cocky about it, because I got you too. Don't even dream about going anywhere."

In no time, I heard that heavy sleep breathing. I knew I didn't have to carefully ease out of the bed because she wasn't going to wake up. I leaned on my elbow a little while longer. In bed or out of the bed, I was "on the job," watching over my baby. When I felt I had gazed long enough, I left the low-light lamp on and left the room without making any noise. But I was still attached, connected by unending love.

I started fast-forwarding the game video tape so I could begin watching at the second half. Meanwhile I cracked open the front door to see how the snow storm was doing. The snow was still coming down. I closed the door fast because the "hawk" was trying to get in my house, so it didn't make sense to shovel my steps tonight. The familiar sounds of a car stuck and spinning its wheels in the ice-packed snow could still be heard from the outside. I stopped the tape, fixed a "Jack and Ginger," and placed Cyn's unfinished steak back into the oven to get the red out the way I liked it. I always complained that I gained weight and she stayed slim because I had to finish off her food to keep from throwing my money away.

Another freezing, snow-blown night in the Windy City. Loving times for some and lonely times for some others. I was one of the lucky ones. I had my game tape, a nice drink, good food, and a pretty woman lying in my bed. Most lovers have their favorite times to be together. Mine was on cold winter nights in January and February. Those nights accentuated my feelings of togetherness and having somebody. They were like being snowed in together. I really loved a snow storm; the cold, the blackness, and especially the noisiness of the wind. I liked hearing that tumultuous howling slamming on my roof and shaking my bedroom window panes. I thought of it as a wind chorus playing on my windowsill. The wind chorus played and sang for us while we were warm, snuggling, and our love for each other was overflowing. The wind played something melodious, loving, and sentimental because the sound of the wind would soar like an overture of strings... then soon quieted in hushed, whispering tones which were hymnal, jazzy, and blues-like.

I guess it's true that everything must change and all good things come to an end. But nowhere in my worst nightmare did I think it would end the way it did. I remembered those fears that I had when my life was the sweetest. Fears about all good things coming to an end too soon; a feeling that our love was too good to last into our golden years. We were newlyweds when she became sick. After so many years of being a bachelor, I was enjoying being married, calling her my wife, and planning things together as husband and wife. I was still getting a rush from calling her on the job and getting that recorded message in that sweet voice, "This is Cindy Gamble, formerly Cindy Lewis. I'm not at my desk now; will you please leave a message?"

When she first became sick, I wondered if we did something wrong to offend God. What could we have done to deserve this? My love, my sweet bride left in December, and in January and February of 1994 winter returned to Chicago with a vengeance. I thought winter was angry at me for mocking it, for taunting it with so many loving winter nights with Cindy. It seemed colder and filled with more falling snow than previous winters. It seemed that there were extra hours of darkness that I just had to bear. What else could I do? I didn't bear it as gracefully as I would have liked, but I got through. Still, I must say for those who have not gone through a great loss, to strengthen yourself spiritually for life is equally unfair. I didn't want to become one of those people that suffered a great loss and became super religious all of a sudden. People actually resent these sufferers telling others they should get closer to God. I don't plan on crusading. I'm content to let people find the healing power of religion in their own time. But for me nothing else could help me but praying and becoming closer to God. If I were closer before this great tragedy in my life, I would have experienced a lesser number of midnight hours grieving and begging, "God, please help me."

Goodbye Wind Chorus

Wind chorus
quit my windowsill and retreat
across the Great Lake's shore,
the joy you brought on snowy
nights don't live here anymore.

halt the aria of strings,
leave the brass unblown,
the wind's just the wind again
its melodies are unknown.

don't ever say her name again
grace, feminality have flown,
the name we
whispered softly in the storm

is written on a gray headstone.

don't play our song, don't hum
along, you and I are through,
your wispy, sentimental sounds
were only meant for two.

goodbye wind chorus,
forget everything of her and me
she has walked into the light,
don't haunt my sweet memories
of those precious snowy nights.

return to me as a gusty breeze
on a scorching hot summer day,
and turn into a hurricane and
blow my depthless sadness away.

JOY: SPIRIT ON THE LOOSE

My Church Lady

Sometimes I hear love songs that remind me of those first exciting months of dating Cynthia. There are other songs that bring sweet memories of various years of us being together. But sometimes I hear church songs that I've never heard before, and they bring on strong memories of Cynthia. The growth in my own spirituality is partly responsible for that, but it's mainly my last impressions of Cynthia as a very spiritual woman.

When we started dating in 1975, religion was not the dominant force in her life, as it became after she was invited to the Apostolic Church of God in 1984. In previous years, she had been an Episcopalian, and she attended St. Edmunds Church. I went with her and her kids to a Christmas midnight mass at St. Edmunds once. Throughout the years, I dropped her off at several of her girlfriend's churches. But other than being invited to Apostolic by a friend, I don't know the other factors that led her to the church and her greater spiritual awareness.

I can't talk about Cynthia's growing spirituality in total isolation. We were soulmates, and what she did affected me. She literally led me back to the church. In our worst hours of need, she taught me how to pray. When I recite the Lord's Prayer today, I can hear her voice reciting in duet with mine, as we did during the great storm. So I'm not just being narcissistic, but hopefully giving some insight into a parallel process that touched both of us. A difficult life is the great recruiter for bringing people to the altar, but we're also influenced to seek God during the best of times.

Cynthia joined the Apostolic Church in 1985. I believe she experienced a spiritual joy over the years that I probably will not be able to experience. She had spiritual joy, and she had us. I have spiritual joy, but I don't have her anymore. I attend Apostolic Church of God regularly these days. Initially, my primary purpose in going was for healing. Every Sunday at Apostolic, the Spirit is on the loose, and besides feeling the Spirit, I strongly feel Cynthia's presence there. When I'm moved by a song I know Cynthia would have loved, I always wish that she were by my side. And when our Bishop gives moving sermons, it always reminds me of the times I had picked her up from church, and she told me, "Bob, you should have heard the Bishop today."

From 1985 on, I drove and picked Cyn up from church practically every Sunday. I didn't attend church in general, but I attended with Cynthia more times than I ever had since I had lived in Chicago. We were married in the Apostolic Church of God in August 1992. I was on my way to becoming a church man when we were married. I had promised her I would attend church with her at least once a month. Like a lot of other guys, my Sunday afternoons were spent at the altars of two different trinities, the NBA and the NFL. But the times I attended Apostolic with Cyn, the experience left a favorable impression on me. First, the service had a set starting time and ending time. That alone was something different from my early days in church in Alabama.

Since I didn't attend church much before, I believed a lot of myths about the black church. But after my first visit, I looked at the church differently; it was not just an escapist institution as I had envisioned it over the years. I believed that the troubles in the black community were so devastating they resulted in the proliferation of liquor stores, storefronts, and a multitude of other churches virtually on every other block. The weak men escaped through the bottle, and the good people escaped through the church. I found that the message in the church was not all doom and gloom. They were not singing a lot of sad songs and talking about dying all the time. It was an upbeat place of joy and love. Although we all have difficulties in life, it wasn't a place peopled only by escape artists reeling from unending hard times. It was clear that life was good for many. They were there to thank God for the things He had done for them, and they were praising God for current blessings.

It took no time for another big myth I believed in to be rebuked — that the church membership consisted of lonely women who didn't have a man, and found a substitute man in Jesus. I recalled this was one of the assertions in the popular book of the 1960s by Eldridge Cleaver, *Soul on Ice*. I'm sure he didn't start the myth. It had existed years before him, and it was a rather widespread belief among the non-church-going male population.

Of course, some female church members are lonely. There are lonely men and women in every large institution. And there may be more women in church than men, but that can't be explained by simply slapping a lonely label on them. Cynthia was there and she wasn't lonely and without a man. Like her, a lot of women had boyfriends and husbands that just didn't attend church on a regular basis. From the first day I attended, I didn't see or sense this alleged loneliness. I was struck immediately by women there who were happy, fulfilled, and service-oriented. There were progressive, career, and professional women everywhere I looked at Apostolic, and I figured it was the same case in most churches. Also, even though I was in church and I was with my soulmate, I couldn't help but notice all of the good-looking women in attendance. They were looking good, dressing sharp, wearing fur coats, and driving big cars. I told Cyn once, "Well babe, I don't have to worry about you catching one of those fast deacons up in there.

You have a lot of competition."

"Oh, you've noticed all of the pretty women we have in our church. They're highly spiritual and highly intelligent, too."

"Right, the last Sunday I was in there with all those pretty women I couldn't concentrate on the sermon. The devil was right in there distracting me."

She laughed, "That's how he works." Then quickly added, "Baby, you got your woman right here, and don't you forget it."

I could see why Cynthia had chosen this church for regular attendance over the many others she had attended throughout the years. I wasn't judging the church from a knowledge of its denominational doctrines, but from what I knew of Cynthia. She was spiritual, but also attracted by intelligence, organization, focus, and service. She was in her element: a large church full of intelligent people, and there were many different ministries for her to choose to work with. Cyn was very service-oriented. She was bound to be more involved in the church than simply attending services every Sunday. Cyn's sorority, Delta Sigma Theta, was also service-oriented. She took the time to learn a new reading method so she could tutor in an adult reading program of her sorority.

As Cyn became more involved in the church, I knew she wanted me to become involved too, but her main focus was concentrating on raising her own level of spirituality. She got both of her children to join the church, and she understood that getting a grown man to join was something different. She didn't know it, but I had planned on going and looking over the church for myself, because I realized that churches are strong social institutions. We would be out at different places, and every once in a while some church guy would walk up being all friendly. He would call out her name, preceeded by "Sister," of course, and give her a tight hug while fervently announcing, "Praise the Lord."

That was supposed to put the boyfriend's mind at ease. He wasn't just a male; he was a church man. But I could look at the guy and instantly tell that he was probably weak on tithing and strong on fornicating. So, when you have a good-looking woman without your ring on her finger, it's a good policy to "break up" into church with her occasionally. It's not about not trusting her; it's all done for her. A boyfriend making himself known saves her from that stigma of being perceived as a lonely woman with no man. Also, it spared her from unnecessary "hits" while she was in a spiritual mood. All right, I'll say it. To a much lesser degree, it's also me saying, "This woman is taken! Praise the Lord!"

I guess getting a woman's mate to church is a problem for many spiritual women, married or unmarried. It was a dilemma for Cynthia. However, she knew I was a believer, I had been raised in the church, and I had a Christian conscience. She would occasionally mention my need for spiritual growth, and I think she had an idea on how to bring this about. She didn't try to recruit me through quotations of Scripture and what a stronger spirituality had done for her. She did want me to attend church, as often as she could get me to go and get to know her Bishop.

Cyn told me, "You'll like our Bishop." She kept emphasizing that I would like this man. She didn't say that I would like his sermons, but that I would respect him and his intellect. She knew that men judge the messenger first, as opposed to judging his message. She knew for sure that I did this a lot; I was just being a typical male. The preacher a man followed had to have leadership qualities that men instinctively recognize in other men. Men sense leadership abilities in other men very early in life, starting with our childhood days on the playground. I'm not just talking about the toughest guy in the neighborhood, but a natural-born leader of men. This instinct follows us through organized sports, the military, and on the job.

I knew about Bishop Brazier as an activist in civil rights

and neighborhood improvement organizations, and those were favorable impressions for me. For a couple of Sundays, I checked him out as a man and not as a preacher. But on those two Sundays, I sensed his leadership abilities, he had an apparent intellect and integrity. The third time I went to church with Cyn, I started listening carefully to what he had to say about the Bible. Because of the way men and women are raised, there's a difference in being a fisherman of men and a fisherman of women. Of course, I know that "fisherman of men" as quoted from the Bible was a general term for men and women, or for all "mankind." (It's hard to get away from sexist terms, isn't it?)

It was obvious to me that Cynthia's growing spirituality was going to change some aspects of our relationship. I didn't anticipate any problems because there was no doubt in my mind that this growth would be for the better. I didn't figure it would be any radical changes in our lives. I thought our moral lives were comparable, or even superior to many of the Christians I knew who were in church every Sunday. In general, men like their women to be religious and involved in the church. Women like the same thing in their men because it gives the illusion, real or imagined, of dealing with a moral person. I think that church people are more moral. They're not perfect — free of sin — but they're trying to recognize what sin is.

I didn't notice a great external change in Cynthia's personality, or her way of acting because of the church. She may not have previously been as spiritual as she was growing to be, but her character was already full of Christian values. She was a moral person and the most compassionate, gentle, and charitable person I've ever known. She was quick to empathize with the problems of others, and she was always available to lend a helping hand.

As Cynthia grew spiritually, she became more and more involved in church activities, or as she put it, "I'm working in the service of the Lord." Putting it in those terms held back my criticism, because I recall thinking, "This church is taking up a lot of my time." She also volunteered to work on various committees. Whatever Cyn was involved in, I also became involved in because I drove her and picked her up from these activities. She once accused me of being resentful of her work in the church. I told her that was ridiculous: "I know you saints want to feel that you are persecuted because of your religious views. You've developed the martyr complex already."

I sat her down and went over her schedule,which included my driving her and picking her up. It started with Sunday morning 11:00 service and sometimes back for the 4:00 service. Some Wednesday Bible studies and Thursday intercessory prayer meetings were also involved. Then there were concerts, retreats, guest speakers, and unscheduled committee meetings. Many of Cyn's Saturday mornings were spent at meetings with special guests at hotels in the Loop. All of this volunteer work went right along with the other things she was doing for her job, sorority, and family. Cyn did not know how to say no. Service was just in her nature, and it was a dizzying pace. Of course, if she could coordinate it, she would hitch a ride with a friend involved in the same activity. But for the most part, driving was part of my dues to pay, and I paid them.

Many Sundays when I would pick Cyn up from church she would be ecstatic about the sermon. "Bobby, you should have heard Bishop today," she often said. I could see her happiness with the church and her religious growth. I didn't get Cyn her first Bible, but I bought her a beautiful Bible with her name etched on it. I bought it at Moody Bibles Book Store. I still made my little digs at her church in a humorous way. I knew it was a Pentecostal, or a Sanctified Church. I expected to see women with no makeup and men with dark blue, Sunday-go-to-meeting suits on at church. But I saw women and men dressed in Gucci and Armani, so I started calling her church members "bourgeoisie holy-rollers."

When I said I didn't notice too much of a change in Cynthia because of the church, I was basically talking about an outer change and a change in our lifestyles. We were not in the streets drinking, gambling, doing drugs, and things of that nature. Still, I really didn't fully understand the inner growth aspects of spirituality. But I could see Cynthia's joy and her not wanting to miss church. She also started sometimes admonishing me for my language. She had changed subtly, but I really shared her joy. It is something very appealing and gratifying to have a spiritual woman in a man's life. Of course, some men speak derisively about a spiritual woman, especially, if they consider her to be fanatical. But even the worst of men have respect for a spiritual, Christian woman who they don't view as being hypocritical.

I loved and respected Cynthia all along, though it soon occurred to me that a growing spirituality brought a different aura to a woman. It's something wonderful that you can see and feel. Sometimes an insecure man becomes uneasy about a woman's growing spirituality. This is not about him loving her less, but a reaction to what he perceives as an erosion of his control. I was very happy for Cynthia. Part of my peace of mind was her not trying to drag me down a road I wasn't ready to travel. I would always say, "I got me a church lady," and she would respond with, "That's exactly right." Sometimes when a religious movie would come on television she would gleefully comment on the Biblical accuracy of the presentation. I didn't become an obstructionist, but for some reason I felt that I should guard against fanaticism or strict fundamentalism. I always pointed out the negatives of a situation concerning Christianity. If we were watching something concerning Native Americans, I would comment on the cruelty of the Spanish Conquistadores in the name of Jesus Christ. I was teaching the novel *Things Fall Apart* by Chinue Achebe in my Afro-history class, so I would talk about Christian imperialism. Those times when she might have disagreed with another church's approach in favor of "what we believed," I would caution her about becoming too sectarian. "Look Cyn, don't get into that 'my church or denomination is right and all of the others are wrong.'"

But I was much more encouraging than critical of her faith because it was obvious our relationship was being strengthened, and it gave her a power to deal with life problems.

I had heard that Pentecostal churches were "marrying" churches. This didn't bother me much because I figured that Cyn and I would get married some day anyway. It was all just a matter of time, and that time would solely be determined by us. But Cyn's growing spirituality brought about changes in her thinking that called for an adjustment in our relationship. She would go on church retreats that lasted at least a few days. When she returned, she was on a spiritual high, strengthened and bubbling over about the speakers and the message. I was happy for her even though she was always on the go with the church and other activities in her life, and I thought she needed to rest more. I would tell her that I thought she was tired, God was everywhere, and I thought she should rest this Sunday. She said I didn't understand. She loved going to church, didn't want to miss going, and it made her feel better when she went. At the time, I really didn't understand the joy of being at a church service as I do now. At the time, I understood that my lover was a tired woman. I wanted to take care of her body, but she wanted to take care of her body and her soul.

Phonycation

A few months before we were married, Cyn and I had our first serious clash over her growing spirituality. She had just returned from a religious retreat when she brought up the subject in a roundabout manner. The issue was about fornication, and though the word "fornication" was never mentioned, I knew instantly what the conversation was about. Marriage was never mentioned either, but it's generally known that in the eyes of "marrying churches," marriage is the solution for the act of fornication. The logic of this thinking has always escaped me. Is sinning — fornicating — a qualification for marriage? Is marriage so insignificant that it's an ex post facto punishment for fornicating? Anyway, I don't know how long she had been thinking about the subject, but I didn't like it, and I put on a show. My approach was a mixture of heretical defiance, male chauvinism, and ghetto logic. I referred to the issue as "phonycation" instead of fornication.

From the first night we discussed this issue and throughout the following weeks, my arguments with Cyn were strictly doctrinal disputes, as opposed to arguments of my being against marrying her. In my mind, getting married to Cyn one day when the time was right was as certain as the sun rising. Our kids were virtually grown and ready to be on their own. I hadn't said anything yet, but I was feeling more and more that the right time for marriage was very near.

Over the years I had made a lot of mistakes in our relationship concerning the approach to various matters, but I'm going to place this tactical error on Cynthia. If only she had just said something very romantic and rhetorically splendid like, "Bob, we've been going together for almost 16 years; it's time for you to piss or get off the pot."

I wouldn't have helped but be touched and moved to say, "Baby that's the prettiest proposal I've ever heard; I accept."

Instead, she opted to be ecclesiastical.

If one of the partners in a couple is spiritual and the other isn't, or is not as spiritual, it's really not wise to approach the other from a strict spiritual point of view. To me, it seemed like her argument for our getting married was not her idea. And what did fornication mean to me? I knew it was not one of the Ten Commandments; maybe it was something doctrinal. But whatever the true intent of sexual relations, it wasn't meant to be an excuse to get married.

I thought the concept of fornication was denominational, like the fact some Pentecostals don't wear jewelry or makeup. The Catholics aren't supposed to eat meat on Fridays during Lent, the Muslims don't eat pork, and the Hindus don't eat beef. Of course, the poor chicken is at the mercy of them all. A man can drink moderately in Christendom; it's my understanding that champagne was first made by a Catholic priest. Though Muslims can't drink alcohol, a Muslim male can legally have three wives in his bed outside of the U.S., so he doesn't really need a drink. And the laws of Judaism and Christianity dictate that you can't have sex with your girlfriend unless you have gone through the vows of Holy Matrimony. These vows are exchanged either in church where people gather to pray or Chicago's City Hall, where politicians gather to prey and occasionally pray.

You can't win with all of these religions and their different denominations. For breakfast on a Friday morning, I might want some smoked sausage, and I want a steak for lunch. I want some pork, beef, or fish for dinner, and a cocktail along with the meal. I want to go out with my pretty woman in my automobile, not in a horse-drawn wagon. I want her to have her face on and wearing the jewelry that I bought her. And it's usually my intention to do what's natural instinct and top off this marvelous evening of good food and drinks with great sex. I've broken rules of various Christian denominations and at least one great revelation in four different religions. What is wrong in one isn't wrong in the other. Of course according to each sect, each received its instructions directly from God. Anyway, all I wanted to do was love my woman and do what was natural. All of these various religions, sects, and denominations should hold a true interfaith ecumenical summit meeting. Their main theme should be "Coordination and Implementation of Revelations and Denominational Regulations for the Prevention of Having a Good Time."

I thought the issue of fornication was ridiculous to be discussing at our ages and coming at that late stage in our relationship. Just looking around at the many husbands cheating on wives, wives cheating on husbands, and sexual perversions in America, how could a loving union of two soulmates be wrong? I attacked with, "Wait a minute! This is not a serious discussion, is it? I know you must be embarrassed even bringing up a subject like this."

I knew that sometimes the church forces a person to take a stand against what their common sense tells them, especially concerning some doctrines that may not be completely outdated but were written when times were much less complex.

"Be for real, Cyn. I can't believe you have allowed the church and some speaker at a retreat to convince you that we're wrong for expressing our love for each other."

She said, "Bobby I'm serious. I want to grow stronger in my faith. I want to have a closer relationship with God."

"I really can't believe this. You sound like somebody who would have followed Jim Jones."

I really felt as though I had been broadsided. I had supported her and pushed her to follow her interest in her church life. I used to say all the time with pride, "I've got me a Church Lady." And I would take her wherever she wanted to go for church matters. Having sex without being married was something I could see as an issue in high school, but we were two divorcees with grown children. I really got angrier at the church than at Cyn. I was thinking that this issue didn't make sense to morally argue about when you think about all of the problems in the world, and the church was still preaching against something as natural as making love by two consenting adults. I know that sex should be regulated, especially for teenagers. I'm also against all forms of perversion, but we were two normal, grown people that were soulmates. I didn't take the subject seriously.

What does a person do when they realize the one they love is going through a serious religious crisis or transformation? It had caught me off guard, but everything soon sank in. Cyn thought things out and wouldn't have mentioned the subject if she wasn't serious. The problem for me was to take it seriously, and I did eventually. It didn't matter what I believed. It was true for her and, at the least, I had to respect that. My common sense told me that a person should always try to support a lover in their search for spiritual growth, but it's not always easy. It's much easier to disagree about the issue of eating meat on Fridays. There are a lot of religious rituals couples can disagree on and can do separately, but sex involves both members. Still, I definitely didn't want to be the ultimate obstructionist for Cyn; one who continues to try and undermine what another person truly considers a quest to save their soul or get closer to God. She knew she had found something wonderful and had wanted to share it with me.

As I have grown spiritually over the years, I can look back and see and better understand which direction God was taking us at a particular time. I know that Cyn and I would have gotten married one day, but unlike God, I didn't know how much time she had left on this side. Now I believe that everything that happened to us was not from our personal timetable, but from the timetable of One who knows all.

When I could plainly see that Cyn was serious, I instinctively wanted to help her, but I still didn't accept the elimination of fornication as the true will of God. I kept thinking about different biblical interpretations... like the slave holders who had used an interpretation of the Bible to justify slavery. They said that black people were children of Ham, or Canaan, on whom Father Noah had laid his famous curse: "And he said, Cursed be Canaan; a servant of servants shall he be unto his brethren." (Genesis 9:25)

I knew that Christendom is full of self-serving interpretations, revisionist revelations; and the sin of fornication, as I saw it, was a denominational interpretation. But Cyn believed in it so I wanted to compromise. I responded one night, "Cyn, you know I don't believe in this, and I don't think the average normal couple can go through with it over a period of time. However, I'm willing to experiment with this charade if for no other reason than to show you that this is abnormal, pure and simple."

I didn't make any advances to try to prove anything because just talking about fornication is enough to turn a man off, period. I mean it really gave me a totally bland feeling about my woman, whom I always thought exuded glamour and sexuality. I looked over and felt as though I was in bed with Aunt Jemima, bandanna and all. Talking about putting a damper on sleeping together, that was it. I felt like this once glamorous thing, this pretty woman whom I stared at while she slept, had on 100 hair rollers, blue face cream, some thick flannel pajamas with feet on them, and her teeth in a glass on the nightstand. I was thinking that this fornication thing was a good thing for then because the way I was feeling, I couldn't have gotten it up if I had to.

More days passed without sex than I thought would,

due in large part to my deflated libido. Anyway, one night we found ourselves lying face to face just fighting for the same air. And everything about her that had drawn me to her, made me love her, and kept me by her side for over 16 years came down on me. The scent of her hair, the light in her eyes, and her moist, Nubian lips brought to my mind that hit song by Luther Ingram, "If Loving You is Wrong, I Don't Want to be Right."

In a whisper, I said, "This is hard, isn't it?" She nodded yes. All that night, I was thinking "I'm going to have to make her Mrs. Gamble just to get my hot mama back." I started thinking that after all of those years maybe it was the time. "Gamble, what the hell are you fighting? You know you want to marry the woman, and you're too much of a procrastinator to pick a date yourself. Go ahead and ask her."

The next day I asked her in a roundabout way. My intent was that her answer would actually end up being her asking me. I didn't have a religious objection to sex while not married.

"Cyn, do you think it's time for us to get married? I've been thinking that maybe it is."

I expected her answer to be something like, "I think it is baby. Sure, let's get married."

But she said, "Are you sure that's what you want?"

"That's not the answer I expected, Cyn. You're acting like I'm begging."

She pulled my head and gave me a smack kiss. "Aren't you?"

"No, I just threw out the question. That kiss was your way of begging me."

"Bobby you just can't come right out and say you want to marry me, can you?"

"Cyn... I wanna make your most perfect fantasy come true."

With a funny look, a sigh, then an arrogant smile, "OK

baby, I accept your heartfelt plea." And that was that.

There was no doubt in my mind that the issue of fornication had brought this on. I was still sort of pissed-off at the church; I was thinking it had stolen my thunder. I just didn't want the decision of when we would get married to go down this way. It felt as though it was not my idea. I had been pushed into it by some outdated concept. After 16 years it should have strictly been my show. What did those shepherds in the Bible know about being romantic? They probably had arranged marriages and didn't live in a world-class city where things like proposals are done over dinner and champagne. Most churches don't excel at "Do this." They excel at "Don't do this."

I said later on, "Cyn, you know I wouldn't marry a woman just so we can make love. I want to make that perfectly clear."

She said, "I didn't ask you to marry me at all, and specifically so we could make love."

"Isn't that the whole concept behind fornication? Isn't marriage supposed to make it right?"

"That's the Word. It's not my Word, but I try to live by it."

"But you've known for a long time I couldn't see my life without us together, and I always knew that we would be married someday."

"I felt the same way for a long time, too, so what's your point?"

"Now you don't understand. I feel like I had a Scripture shotgun held to my head. I didn't want anything like fornication to be anywhere near our decision to get married. I wanted to be more romantic."

"Bobby, it's 1992. You had a whole lot of years to buy a diamond, plan a trip, send roses, or whatever."

Now that we had the marriage ball rolling, she felt much better about things. She took Aunt Jemima out of my bed and put Glamour Girl back in, so I felt much better too.

There wasn't much planning to do for our wedding because it was going to be a very small affair. It definitely was going to be in church, and overall I felt really good about it. It was like something in my life that I knew would happen someday, but I didn't know when. I felt in no way trapped. It was sort of a relief. After my initial outbursts, I was thinking that the church was smarter than I was. It had done me a big favor by giving me that little push to marry my soulmate, the love of my life.

We went to the courthouse in Markham, Illinois to get a marriage license. I recall us sitting in the office waiting, and we were the oldest couple there. We were commenting on how cute all the other couples looked, and I felt that we were the only ones there that really knew what we were getting into. I wanted to wish all of them good luck, because I knew what it meant to be young and starry-eyed, but how in a few years a couple can end up hating each other.

For the next few weeks we shot a lot of jabs at each other: "All right, Cyn, you know I think that education spoils a good woman. And don't think that carrying a corporate credit card cancels out your subservient position in this merger. Don't even buy Jiffy corn bread mix. I expect all of my food to be prepared from scratch."

She said, "Baby, I didn't tell you, but I'm planning on turning the kitchen into a den."

So for weeks we went back and forth with jabs at each other. It was the chauvinist vs. the feminist, and it went on and on.

I've condensed what happened. The beginning of the discussion of marriage, covered maybe eight months before we were married. I guess she was sick even back then; something evil inside of her was growing. I believe that God in his infinite wisdom had brought us together as husband and wife. I was to take care of her as her husband during the great storm. I would have been right by her side as her soulmate, but being husband and wife was different.

I said early on that not saying "I do" and our not living together were the reasons for the high level of romanticism and long years of happiness that Cyn and I shared. I'm not backtracking now by saying that was not true. I don't know all of the answers. But if I was wrong, it still did not separate me from the love of God. I have sweet memories of picking out the plain gold ring and the happiness of our wedding day. I hear her voice when I called her on the job. When she answered, I said romantically, "I would like to speak to Mrs. Robert Gamble."

And sweeter than sweet she would reply, "Speaking, this is she... heyyy baby!"

I've been blessed because there's one thing for sure, and it haunts me to even think about it. If I had not married the woman I had loved so well and for so long, if I had not stood at the altar before God and taken her as my wife, it would have been my life's biggest regret; one I would have mulled over and suffered about until the day I died. I almost missed it, but I didn't. Thank you sweet Jesus.

Wedding Day

A splash of dog days sun
tangerine, radiant, warm
city noises, city scenes
        people
going about their business,

my son, her daughter
        a tiny
gathering of friends

"finally," "it's about time,"
"after all these years,"

giant sanctuary, lofty ceiling,
        empty
row after row of mahogany pews.

Light Is Softly Reflecting

off her white linen suit,
her hair streaked with silver,
        in her
sparkling and beautiful eyes

she's rampant femininity,
hot-blooded steamy grace.

I do, I will, I love you,
        we're
blessed, bonded, forever.
Ah shucks! The girl is mine!

Diva

a flower, a butterfly
complicated and pretty
she's an acquisitor by
    a smile,

interpreter of her man's
    transparency

    clairvoyant of
his desires and essence

    she holds
the title on herself
but if a man's got it
    together,
she is giving, loving,
    passionate

    the woman's
quintessential female
a conductor of heat
bouquet of pheromones

she's a diva undeniably

  the lady
expects preferential
  treatment,
and she's gonna get it.

Abduction & Possession

I've captured a butterfly
my grasp is a gentleness
I'd never mastered before
  that's because the
butterfly has a delicacy
  I've never felt.

  In my heart a
flower has sprouted and it
radiantly blooms in my soul,
  only a
fine-crystal vase designed
for a singular yellow rose
  knows how I feel.

I Do, I Will

I reminisced about the early days on my way over to the church to get married. A couple of weeks earlier I had said to myself, "Wait a minute… getting married? Gamble, of all things, what the hell are you excited about?" I really couldn't understand why I was feeling so good about it. Maybe it was because I didn't expect any changes from what we had been doing all along. I had realized that I wanted to be with her for the rest of my life, but I had been afraid that marriage would mess that up.

Sometimes we would throw the question out in a playful manner. She would always say, "Let's secretly get married but continue to live apart like we're doing."

I would always come back with, "We're already married."

One night we performed the marriage ceremony that black slaves invented because they were forbidden by law to be married. I placed a broom on the floor, and we jumped over it. But Cyn would always say, "That's not good enough."

Once I replied to that, "Why not? Oh… you want us to go down to City Hall, get a license, and let the white man tell us that we're married like in slavery days."

And she said, "That's only part of it. I wanna see my name on your pension, insurance, see you paying the bills, and handing over the rent check, that's marriage."

The day had finally arrived, and I had a number of

mixed feelings, but a lot of things were going right with my life at the time. My boy was in the city college. I had high hopes that he would finish and transfer to a four-year university. Cynthia's boy was in his second year of law school at the University of Michigan, and her daughter was to leave for Southern University in Louisiana in August. In February I had given Cynthia a nice birthstone and diamond ring that she really loved. She would be watching her finger as we drove around, and it really did dress up her beautiful hand. There wasn't going to be any radical changes in our lives. She stayed at my house a lot anyway, and our lives were already very much intertwined.

I thought the wedding would be in one of the many smaller rooms in the church, but our group of friends gathered in the large sanctuary, which swallowed up our small party. In the church I was loose and feeling content as we would glance at each other while she conversed with one of the church ladies about the preacher or whatever. I was content to just sit chatting with my friends and let her take care of what needed to be taken care of, because I felt it was her church and her territory.

We were in place in front of the minister, Pastor Larry Martin, and my friend, James Shelton, was on my side, her girlfriend, Terri Vanderjack, was on her side, and her daughter, Crystal, was giving her away.

A wave of loving feelings swept over me when I looked at Cyn. She had on a white linen short-sleeved suit dress. She had a bouquet which looked like gardenias to me. With her hair swept back and up, I thought she was a classic beauty. Her hair was streaked with silver, but her face looked the same as the day I met her. I felt a little like I was marrying a stranger. Even though, I believed I really knew her through all of the years, I was certain of only one thing: she was joy!

Our honeymoon was going to be our trip to Baton Rouge to take things to her daughter who had just enrolled in college. Neither of us had been to New Orleans or Bourbon Street, and we looked forward to it.

We were married on the first day of August and Cyn, Jason, and I drove to Southern University in the middle of August with a lot of clothes and provisions for Crystal who was already there. We had a great time eating at several restaurants in Baton Rouge and had a really great time listening to jazz on Bourbon Street. We drove to New Orleans twice and toured the city. Jason and Cyn always liked trying different cuisines, so we ate at many different places. We really had a grand time, and New Orleans was tops on our list to visit again as soon as possible.

When we left Louisiana we cut across the gulf area of Mississippi heading for Montgomery, Alabama, my hometown. We were in a hurry to leave Louisiana because of Hurricane Andrew. We stopped in Montgomery to see my mama and my brother, Renard. My mama was ecstatic that Cyn and I were finally married. Jason was going into his second year of law school and I always introduced him with, "We now have us a lawyer in the family." We headed to Atlanta but first we stopped at Tuskegee University. When describing myself, one of the things I say off the top is, "I'm a Tuskegee man." I was giving Jason his black college tour. We had already toured five black college campuses and would visit five more in Atlanta. Jason had finished his undergraduate work at MIT. He was at Michigan for his law degree, so I wanted to make sure he got a chance to see as many historical black colleges as he could.

I had three brothers — Billy, Harold, and Alonza — and their families all living in Atlanta. We stayed overnight at Alonza's, the bachelor house, and the rest of the family came to us. They all welcomed Cyn to the family as the new Mrs. Gamble.

There was something glorious about this trip. I told Cyn over and over in the next few months how much I had real ly enjoyed it. Being newlyweds can explain part of it, but it was much more. If you're not spiritual, you may want to dismiss my theory, but as I have grown spiritually, it's crystal clear to me that this was one of those mysterious ways that the Lord works in.

Marriage was smooth sailing for us, just uneventful bliss. Most things about our lives remained the same, but there was this feeling of being much closer, and I can't recall a single dispute about anything. Cyn's life was still more complicated than mine. Technically, she still had two residences and still got off the bus from work in front of her building. She would still see after her mother, cook for her some days, or we would get her something to eat. Both of her children were still in school, and Cyn was still the head of the household. I guess the main difference in our relationship was that we stayed together every night. We still ate the big meals for Thanksgiving and Christmas at her apartment.

I'd always tried to make Cyn's life easier, but you can imagine that her situation was difficult. I ordered most of the Thanksgiving and Christmas dinners precooked because a lot of families do that now. Working women don't have time to spend all day and night cooking like they used to do in the old days. I didn't expect a working woman to be sweating over the stove all evening, and we had our plans to redo my house (or our house) now. We were going to redecorate the whole place and maybe sell in three years. We were going around to stores and picking out our wall colors, carpet colors, and deciding what furniture we would get rid of and what we would buy. The planning for everything was a lot of fun. I just had to make sure things were not too feminine.

I didn't think that marriage would make a difference as to how I felt about Cynthia, but I was wrong. I was surprised that I felt much closer and loved her even more. "I do" took our love to a higher level. I told her, "If I had known that marriage would have made me this happy, I would have accepted your proposal a long time ago." But it was still taking a while for us to stop thinking independently.

For the last year and a half or so, Cyn had lived under the shadow of her company downsizing. That's rough for anybody in management, and especially for female single parents. I had always made it as clear as I could that we were soulmates, and if push came to a shove, she should take the best buyout deal. We would proceed together from there. When we were married, it took some of the pressure off her. I guess to a woman, a man can say anything, but the marriage paper is putting it in writing and is binding.

We had always said that we could never do each other's job. I knew my job was hard, getting harder, and so was hers. She would bring home big books every night. I would drop her off or go to the Loop to work with her on Saturday mornings, and would pick her up between eight and ten at night. Ameritech paid well, but the employees really had to work hard for it. My pet name for the company was "Massa Bell" instead of "Ma Bell."

These were blissful times; nothing could stop our growing love for each other. Life is tough, but when you have somebody who loves you and somebody to come home to, you can deal with most anything. For our first six married months we were still on our honeymoon.

A CAPTIVE IN THE CAMP OF GRIEF AND SADNESS

Courting Ms. Sadness

It's one of the
last things I wanted to do… but
it feels like I've fallen in love
with sadness;
it feels like we're mated, opiated,

floating together and
sometimes it's a strange pleasure
reminiscing and gazing
at beautiful rosy horizons through
watery eyes.

I can't say why, but there seems
to be something sweet, alluring
about melancholy
and she does cradle me, touching
where no other woman can.

Why is sad music so much prettier?
I revel in the lamenting-sounds of
rising and falling strings, long for
pathos, gathering and escaping from
softly touched piano keys;
they sweep me and they sleep with
my precocious self-pity.

still… from another side of me,
I'm praying that we'll part soon
because sadness is a lover, a woman
that has to be jilted.

I must be just lying with her and
using her, for I'm
needing, waiting on somebody else;
Ms. love and happiness to hurry along.

By Myself

I can't shake it,
I've tried getting out of the way
walking fast, running,
going places, hiding,
it follows me to places where nobody
else can go, I just can't escape it
Somebody help me!

It's not just swarming in my dreams
or like a fanfare in a quiet chamber
of my mind,
it's with me in radiant sunlight
at crowded malls, at Soldier Field

It's in my head, it's in my bed

the feeling's pervasive, permeating,
I've had it since the day she left
Somebody help me!
can't help feeling… I'm by myself.

Beauty Unrequited

When she was
warm and present in my life,
a spectacular day
was spiritual, accentuated.

Posing
for the shutter or the canvas
Ms. Nature expressed herself
in beautiful technicolor days
filling me with

lines, rhymes, loving feelings,

and I was swept
soaring like cottony seeds in
stiff Windy City breezes.

Now a perfectly beautiful day
only accentuates my feelings
of loneliness.

Clouds scattered
across a vast twilight sunset
are warm and cool pastel colors.

They're
streaking, fibratus, splashing,
dancing sensually

looking like a chorus line,

and crepuscular rays of the sun
fan the horizon in
long columns of brilliant light.

The brilliant, heavenly colors
are stunning for so many, but
it's gloriousness wasted on me.

    In my
loneliness colors are trapped,
    like colors
in a prism… in fine crystal,

shining, sparkling, glittering
    but scurrying,
peeking out, wanting to escape.

    They're like my joy,
once saturating, overpowering,
but now, hidden someplace deep
    in my insides.

    The colors
in the prism, in fine crystal,
in a clear, shimmering diamond

are longing… to be released,
I'm longing… to be released,

    longing
for the sight of sheer beauty
    to fill me again with

lines, rhymes, loving feelings.

    Touch me again,
beautiful days, spiritual days,
    I want to be released.

Being a Widower

When we were together as
soulmates
I verbalized and excelled
at captivity philosophy,

just running off my mouth
about how it would be to
be a free man,

"There are plenty of fish
in the sea,"

"There's no one person in
the world for anybody,"

"No one woman can satisfy
a man's total physical
and psychological needs,"

sometimes I thought about
something happening to our
relationship,
specifically, if she found
somebody and just left me,

I figured
sooner moreso than later

I would rebound after the
hurt and eventually top
even her.

Now that
she's gone and I'm alone,
apparently available and
surrounded by
the world pool of women,

the months have gathered
past a year and they're
rolling on,

damn! damn!
it would really help me if
I could back up all of the
chauvinist philosophizing
I used to excel at

in these
uncertain days I feel like
a pitiful excuse for a man,
for the philosophy,
"I can always get a woman
if I really need one."

I know I've got to move on,
I'm trying to,
but my reality is

I just can't let her go.

God help me!
— I still belong to her.

Almond, Cherry, Elderberry

An Indian summer day
walking in the hub of this mighty
beautiful city.
Chicagoans call it "the Loop" and
it's busy, tall, sprawling, noisy
world-class.

I sneaked a kiss, held Cyn's hand
in the Loop for nearly two decades;
she's walking beside me in my head,

for I'm daydreaming
of technicolor days, cool nights,
good times that can never be again.

Skyscrapers emptying
people scurrying out like children
piling into the schoolyard to play,

strolling broad sidewalks
passing summertime, sidewalk cafes
strolling
on silver steel mechanical bridges
over the zig-zagging Chicago River,

Windy City cuties
lovely precious ones of other guys
going to lunch, or window-shopping,
sunbathing, chilling, manhunting,

looking
stylish, sophisticated, and expensive,
blood strands of
Africa, Europe, Asia, and the Islands.

Business finished
basking in the beauty of the day,
admiring the
glass, steel, terra-cotta forest.

Along the river,
walking briskly down Wacker Drive
is where I saw her and though
she was over a block away I still
flinched involuntarily,

from that distance, she looked so
much like Cynthia.

It was
something about the way she moved,
her build, her hair,
I didn't know what to think or do.

from a little less than a block
it was her,

she's closer, other things about
her added to that haunting image.
She wore
gold, a red blouse, medium heels,
and her dark slacks fitted loose,

still, I knew it couldn't be her.

But like
Cynthia her complexion's almond
her lips are cherry and her
eyes are black as an elderberry.

Closer still,
I felt I had pulled myself together
but when I clearly saw her face
rationalism flew away,

love and remembrances
began to rain on this cloudless
airy and beautiful Indian summer day.

/along the river, cars were rounding/
/their horns were loudly sounding/
/and my heart was steady pounding/
/harder and harder in my chest/

Didn't believe my eyes,
on a conscious level I knew better,
I just wanted it to be her so much,
to be
the morning after I had awakened and
everything in the past months were
a long nightmare.

/her complexion's the color of almonds/
/her lips are red like cherries/
/her eyes are round and beautiful/
/and black like elderberries/

Breathing very hard,
I was afraid the people strolling
leisurely around me could hear me.

Feeling lightheaded
but I made up my mind that I wasn't
going to let her catch me staring
unashamedly,

hoping that she slowed, noticed me
        just look my way and
let our eyes meet in a glance;
that will tell me everything I
wanted and needed to know about her.

/will her eyes shine right through me?/
/hi stranger! ...long time no see!/
/will I see the look of love again/
        /shining affectionately on me?/

the breezes are playing in her hair
flapping her silk blouse like a sail
        and a smile came
across her face but it wasn't for me.

maybe she thought back on something
he had whispered lovingly in her ear
        late last night or
very early on this late, summer morn.

/I could feel her sensual presence/
        /it was nothing she did or said/
/it's something arousing in my memory/
        /that's always in my head/

        Almost side by side
I put on a friendly, gentleman's stare,
        that look of familiarity saying we
knew each other or worked for the same
        company.

        That was quick thinking,
        something very innocent
        and unassuming.

        Suddenly!
the thought entered my mind that
maybe she had scoped me already?

was drawn to me as I was to her.

had lightning struck twice?
        why not?
she looked so much like Cynthia
and we were nice-looking together.

        Maybe something
mystical, fate, even supernatural
        would draw her to me
or something alluring, passionate
        and maybe even loving.

/she's close, want to embrace her/
/she looks sweet, want to taste her/
/but I would be afraid to face her/
/if she stopped and touched my hand/

for some reason, I caught her eye,
probably acknowledging my stare as
a compliment like some attractive
        women do sometimes,

but it wasn't even a come-on look,
        nor an erotic look
and nothing near the look of love.

        Barely audible
her lips moved, and she flashed
        a wry smile
she was past me in a split second.

She was
/some lucky guy's pretty woman/
/a sweet thing he wined and dined/
/she looked a lot like my woman/
/that shattered my peace of mind/

/her swagger, a face so familiar/
/a mirage aphrodisiac/
/swished by like a windy city breeze/
/I knew I shouldn't even look back/

Still,
/I turned around and watched her/
/because my heart was in her hand/
/but she didn't know I even existed/
/she belonged to some other man/

/another scene, like another dream/
/reminding me that I'm alone/
but halting
/my slide into the twilight zone/
/I kept moving and heading for home/

/she's heading home to him tonight/
/she's his woman, she's not mine/
/she looked a lot like my baby/
But
/my baby was one of a kind/

And
/her complexion's the color of almonds/
/her lips are red like cherries/
/her eyes are round and beautiful/
/and black like elderberries/

Thinking of Her While Walking With an Orange Sun in Black Naked Trees

in winter
living-things cover themselves
except for most trees because
they become uncovered, leafless,
bareheaded & naked.

I love trees in summer, green,
noisy in a rustling duet with
the wind, but
I also love to watch rows of
tall trees silhouetted bushy,
forestal, stark-naked against
a clear winter sky.

a winter evening sun's golden,
falling fast, changing color,
walking briskly
the trees are moving past me
the sun's dotting in and out
following me
romping in uneven silhouettes
of black naked trees,
ray-blinding, hiding, swelling

a gigantic, burnt-orange sphere
stalled on the horizon
shining faintly, but splendidly
in a melancholic sky, lapis,
tranquil, starkly beautiful in
coral twilight slowly vanishing.

But What Does It Matter?

beauty's always
good company, although sometimes
    what does it matter?

    some nights on the lake
moonbeans shimmer like sequins on
the skirt of a long-legged dancer,
    it was technicolor
and gusty with the Midwestern sun
    struttin' high, maybe
it was a race to Mackinac Island?

it was surely a spectacular sight
rows of circling sailing boats on
    the Great Lake,
their multi-colored sails bloated,
color-scheming the blue horizon

    right behind me on the
western side of Lake Shore Drive
    tall white maples
with leaves green on one side and
    silver on the other,

    unparalleled beauty
in the long row of tall trees as
splendrous leaves are moving like
    swelling ocean waves,
but sometimes what does it matter?

    ain't got nobody to sit
with me and share all the beauty.

Alonea

Late last night, early in the
black morning, my ever-present
deep loneliness became a woman
    and she
crept in the dark into my bed.

She slithered under my blanket
snuggling close behind me,
annoyingly, but calmly
I whispered, "You are not who
    I want you to be."

    Strangely,
her touch had a familiarity
that plays over and over
in my dearest reminiscences.

    I knew
I had smelled her sweet scent,
felt her hot touch and breath,
    when she gently
placed her nipple in my mouth,
I knew I had tasted her before.

    I reveled
in sheer ecstasy for a while
feeling heat made only by two,
    but in no time
as suddenly as they had come
every sensation disappeared,

the sweet scent, heat, taste,
and the breathing were all gone.

My sheet
was unruffled and cold again.
I felt an emptiness in my bed
momentarily, but
faint exhaling, a female scent,
something, somebody reappeared
lying beside me.

I was shaking as I slowly asked,
"Who are you? "Why did you
seduce me with precious memories
that can never be again?"

She answered,
barely audible though cold and
ticklish in my ear saying that
she and I
were wedded now and vowed that
she and I
will always be together while
I'm alive, living on this side.

Then seductively a hot tongue
dotted in and out of my ear
cold lips pressed on my cheek,

and in an utterance revealing
who she is, what I am,
siren-like, nymphal, angelic,
she whispers sweet as licorice

"my name is Alonea,
your name is Alone."

Everybody Else

everywhere I go
they're all I ever see,
lovers strolling
all hugged-up

like we used to be,

lying under a large
beach towel
kissing in the shade
of a cottonwood tree

everybody has somebody
… everybody but me

Coming and Going

yesterday I was driving past
a hospital and started musing
    about things,
pretty things like teddybears
balloons, tiny, pink blankets,
    and festive things
hanging from the ceiling like
    silver-tinsel stars
blue moons, plum-red festoons,

    inevitably I started
musing about flowers, prayers,
    get-well cards
pills, morphine, oxygen-tanks,

    life's antonyms,
all of those things under the
    same roof
but on different floors, wards,

    simultaneously
something's bringing smiles, joy
something's bringing tears, pain
    and we must accept it,

    might as well,
ain't nothing unusual it's just
    life inexorably
scribbling a name in the ledger,
    somebody's coming
    somebody's going.

THE SUN SETTING, BODY STORM RISING

Body Storm on a Red Day in Autumn

Capricious days
of budding autumn are tired so
they shorten themselves but on
this red and windy day the air
wasn't dry, calm, and all of a
sudden became wet and heavy,

the Great Lake
wasn't flat, serene, and all of a
sudden the waves began to swell,
neither
did the blue skies blacken and

the wind didn't
whisper one moment and become
a deafening howl minutes later.

Wish it were so,
but we couldn't run for cover and
there's no hatches to batten down;
wish that there were.

Better if it were
but it wasn't a Kansas twister,
churning the treeless prairie and
splintering large faded-red barns,

nor was it a furious
north Atlantic storm when sailors
tossed and helpless would sing
their hymn to the Eternal Father:

"Oh hear us when we call to thee
for those in peril on the Sea."

    Wish it wasn't so
but it was a body storm raging.

    Nature's
unmerciful and heartbreaking
way of thinning the herd,
revealing only the symptom

that cries wolf year after year.

The body storm's an ancient enemy
    dreaded, feared,

as old as the wedding vows which
on the most loving of days pay
homage to the power of the storm:

"In sickness and in health."

On the blessed day we were married,
sickness unperceived, camouflaged
was advancing silently but

true to its clandestine nature

it allowed us to be happy, to laugh,
make plans and dream of many years
    together.

in October a pleasant chill had
come with the change of seasons
and the Earth ornamented itself

with the technicolor days of autumn.

Blush-red days,
crimson skies and falling leaves
in variant colors of red: auburn
rust, reddish-brown, puce, henna,

and the earth is
birch-tree white, fir-tree green
corn-cob yellow, pumpkin-orange
berry-brown, Lake Michigan-blue.

The late evening sun is halted,

it's coloring windows orangy on
the top 40 floors of gleaming
skyscrapers rising 70 stories
off the midwestern prairie and

the
lakefront's unrestful, blustery,
the wind's
gusting and the water is spraying.

hugged tight, walking hand in hand,
sand and leaves twirled all around
our heads and we covered our faces
momentarily before

lovingly and carefully
I picked twig and colorful, tiny
fragments of leaves from her hair,

barely finished, she sharply tugged
on my coat snapping,
"Hey sweet baby! I love you a lot."

I leaned and kissed her cheek
which had an autumn feeling,
        like
pressing my lips to a large red
apple that's smooth, cold, and dry,

        very much unlike
the sweet, warm and moist feeling
of kissing her cheek just a few
        hot weeks ago.

        The change of
seasons brings different scenes
feelings, modes of expression.
Nature's way of being romantic.

        I looked forward to
an old-fashioned Chicago winter,
gray, freezing, ice and snow storms.

        Walking along
I was daydreaming about the "hawk,"
she and I on a cold winter night
        loving and snuggling, but
though hidden, the storm's raging.

        Nevertheless!
soaked in the bliss of autumn on
this beautiful red and windy day
we had no thoughts, even remotely

about the wounding of the swan
the end of laughter, no more we.
Almighty and merciful God help us!

Happiness in Full Retreat

I was on the job. When you have a difficult job like I had, normally it's an unlikely place, a wrong place, a wrong time for fostering loving feelings... but maybe not. Maybe it's because of the difficulty, the concentration on the tasks blanking out thoughts of my personal life that made those thoughts of her so sweet when they returned to me.

During my lunch period, I made what was to be a quick call to Cynthia just to say hello. I wanted to hear her voice and tell her again that I loved her. Her voice was normal when she answered the phone, but it changed quickly as she recognized my voice. She was quiet, but her voice broke into a distressed tone, on the verge of tears mode.

"Bobby, I discovered a lump on my neck."

I said, "What kind of a lump?"

She replied, still sounding tearful, "I don't know, but Lynn said a lump on your neck is always a bad sign."

"OK, Sweet, are you going to the doctor to have it checked out?"

She said she had an appointment later on that day.

I said, "All right, Baby, let's be positive. Try not to worry. You want me to pick you up from there?"

She said she was going for the appointment, coming back to work, and she would call me later at home.

When we had awakened that morning, it was a day like any other day, but just like that... it was the last day of our happiness. It was a plunge from the great height of loving bliss to an abyss of sadness. And that toll of events would render me being like I am now, one of the loneliest men on Earth.

Cynthia was very knowledgeable about a lot of medical conditions. She had high blood pressure, so she was a regular visitor to the doctor. About two years earlier, she had a scare about her breast which prompted a mammogram. I remember her shaking so bad the night before that I had to hold her as tight as I could practically the whole night. That crisis passed with good results, and it seemed like no time had passed before we were into another crisis. For most of that night, she shook again before falling off to sleep.

Her doctor had quickly scheduled a biopsy. I believe it was the very next day. Meanwhile, we were reading through every book we could get our hands on to gain more information about lumps. Cyn's strong faith gave her reason to search for the best, so she was sort of upbeat when I took her in for the biopsy. She was her old self, friendly and gracious, during the outpatient stay. She talked about how nice everybody was, and it took about three days for the results to come back.

I had gone to work and was already back at home when Cyn called telling me the results of the biopsy; "Bobby, the doctor said it was malignant. I have cancer."

At that moment, everything I had been taught about being a man, about a man doing what a man has to do, abandoned me. I cursed to myself before asking, "What kind?... Where?"

She said that he wasn't sure. She said her doctors would send her to an oncologist. I was completely stunned, but I kept my composure until I hung up. That conversation was the most soul-shaking experience of my life. I took it harder than the news of my father's death in an auto accident, because death is so definitive, and there's nothing anybody could do at that stage.

I had never felt so helpless in my life. My baby had been attacked by cancer. I kept thinking about how she was feeling. She was so compassionate for others that she had a physical reaction to terrible news. How scared must she be?

I thought. Could I do anything, or say anything to console her? For myself, I was thinking that the one person on this Earth that made me the happiest could die. Because I didn't know anything about the disease, I only thought about Cyn dying. I had no idea how much cancer patients suffer, and how much she would suffer. This is the nightmare that lovers deeply in love have always dreaded. That question was upon me: "What will I do without you?"

I knew I had to be strong for my baby, and I was going to be. I was going to do everything that needed to be done in the manner it needed to be done. Like everybody had always advised, I was going to get on top of the situation. I was going to read and amass as much information about the disease as I could. I knew I was going to be a great support for Cynthia. I knew I would help her to pray and would always be there for her to lean on. I couldn't let Cyn see me weak and without faith. I could wear the mask of supreme confidence if that would help Cyn with her positive outlook. But all of that would come later.

For most of my life, sadness was a stranger, and crying was even more of an anomaly. I thought about that short verse of scripture that people relied upon because they couldn't memorize anything longer: "Jesus wept." Still, does crying do any good? I'm a strong man, and I'll do what I have to do as the saying goes. But at that hour, because of the hand life had dealt my baby… all I wanted to do… all I could do… was cry.

Desperate Times

I should have taken a couple of days off from work. I'm pleasant by nature, and acting pleasant and being funny is what my students and co-workers expected of me. But it was a day like I've never had. I knew everything showed on my face, so I tried to be alone as much as possible. Since I had responsibilities and had to work, I planned on making the best of it.

After the shock of the first couple of days, I pulled myself together. Cyn was in a stage where she didn't appear any sicker than she did in the days or years before. But we knew about the cancer now, and that made a world of difference about our lives. Naturally, our first hope was that it was something that could be removed, or be quickly put into remission. Her regular doctor's first job was to turn her over to a cancer specialist, an oncologist. His first job, I believe, was to order fifty million tests. I guess sometimes tests detect things right away, and other times the disease is like an animal that knows it's being hunted. It becomes extremely elusive to all of science's tests and high-tech machinery.

I don't have the inside information on what went on between Cynthia and her doctor. On our first visit to the oncologist, he came out to greet us. I guess he expected both the husband and wife to come into his office for consultation, but Cynthia nixed the idea. She said, "Bob, wait here. I want to talk to the doctor alone."

I was thinking that the way I cried that first day must have her thinking that I couldn't take any bad news. On the way home, I asked her, "Why didn't you want me to come along?"

She replied, "Baby, I'm used to going and talking to the doctor by myself. I know the questions to ask. I'll keep you fully abreast."

I can only guess at the full reasons behind her position, but I know they included keeping the bad news away from me and the rest of her family. Also, we had this independent way of doings things that lingered with both of us even after we were married. We were very quiet on the way back from the Loop to our home, and we didn't say anything once we were in the house either. She sat on one sofa; I sat on the other. I was just going to wait until she decided to change the mood and say something, so we sat there in silence. She had on a very complimentary red turtleneck sweater, and her face was leaning on her hand. She looked sad and worried, but not sick. I was thinking that this has to be the second worst day of her life, but she was still looking very pretty. I said, "Babe, I know this is one of the worst days of our lives, but you're still looking pretty. I wanna take your picture, so we can look back on this day years from now when things are much better. I hope you don't mind?"

She shook her head slightly. I grabbed my camera and took the picture. It was to be a picture we would look at years later, showing how she held up under the strain of way back when. I had absolutely no thoughts whatsoever that this picture would sit atop her brushed-metal casket just ten months later.

I didn't fight her about why I couldn't be in on the sessions with the doctor. It showed our unpreparedness as a unit, and how fast things in our lives had changed. The doctors knew her as Ms. Lewis, because that was her name on all of her medical documents. I really didn't want to be treated like her kids with information being kept away from me, so I told her I could handle what needed to be handled. I felt that she understood that I could.

Tests were really a big part of the treatment, but it seemed like while they were going on, nothing was being done to attack the disease. While we were waiting on the standard chemotherapy, radiation, or surgery treatment to get started, we were looking into any alternative and Eastern treatments. The fight to live is a desperate fight, and living in a world-class city like Chicago gives a person the opportunity to explore alternative medicine without leaving town. We got started right away.

In the next few weeks before Cyn's radiation treatments started, we dived head first into the cancer fighting industry. We read everything we could get our hands on concerning symptoms and types of cancer. We knew that the survival rates for the different cancers varied. We prayed that hers would be a type with the best chance of remission and the longest survival rate. I was not in the meetings with Cyn and her oncologist, but I got my information from her about everything I wanted to know. I believe that she didn't want to ask her doctor point-blank how many months or years she had to live. I could be wrong, but sometimes people just don't want to hear the worst. Also, it's just possible that she didn't want her family or me to deal with the worst news. I remember my heart sinking when she told me that it was inoperable lung cancer. Even with that information, it was her spiritual belief that ultimately only God gives life and takes life, and God can reverse and has reversed much worse situations. Her job was to pray, be positive, and fight for life as hard as she could. She told me on the first day that she didn't mind dying; she only said she didn't want to suffer. She also said, in reference to my sister-in-law who had died from leukemia in 1988, "I can't be like Dot." Dot was very religious and had suffered through her illness with little complaining. It actually ended up that Cyn was a lot like

Dot, a strong spiritual woman, a fighter doing what she had to do, without showing the terror she must have been feeling.

Only once did I hear Cyn ask, "Why did this happen to me?" But she quickly caught herself because she had planned to keep her faith strong; to keep a very positive attitude, as the books and tapes suggested. I kept a positive attitude also, but that question of why her and how it happened haunted me. I'm still wondering today about what part stress played in Cyn's illness, because there were a series of more stressful than normal events in Cynthia's life the three years before her illness. They were really more traumatic than simply being stressful.

It was on a Wednesday evening. I was driving Cyn to a meeting with her committee at church. We always passed right by her best girlfriend Lynn's house to get to the church. "Cyn and Lynn!" I used to always refer to them in a very loud voice. We noticed three police cars parked by her door. Cyn said, "Stop," and I could see that same panicked, worried look on her face that I had seen on occasions for the last months with Crystal. I couldn't find a parking space so Cyn said, "Just let me out here."

I drove about a block up and got a parking space. I was walking back and was almost at the house when Cyn came out of the door walking toward me. I could see her looking stunned and shaken like I had never seen her before. I hurried and asked, "What's wrong Sweetheart?"

Her voiced broke, she was half-crying, but in that state where a person seems too shocked to outright cry. She replied, "Lynn is dead!"

It stunned me. I quickly asked, "What?"

"Roosevelt shot her, and then he shot himself. His body is still in the bedroom."

I hugged her, and we walked back toward my car. She was able to cry by this time. I didn't ask any more questions right away because I was stunned and shaken up, too.

She said, "Take me on to the church."

I accompanied her into the meeting with the other church ladies, and I knew they knew what to say and do to comfort her and her friends in their Christian way.

Cyn's boy, Jason, and I were really worried about Cynthia's reaction during Lynn's wake. Cynthia was to participate in their sorority's (Delta Sigma Theta) ceremony. Cyn held up and did her part well. The next day I was a little slow in getting ready for the funeral. Cyn was impatient, so she left earlier with her son. I sat in a spot in the balcony where I could watch her. At the funeral I didn't get emotional until the end of the service when they were pushing out the casket. When it passed Cyn, she reached out, touched it, and then threw a kiss goodbye. It just hit me that losing a best girlfriend was like losing a family member. Knowing Cyn's personality, I knew that she had been shaken to the core, and there would be some deep mourning for a long time. A part of her world was gone, and I could no longer holler out, "Cyn and Lynn!" Cyn hid the worst of her mourning from me, but she shared it with her other girlfriends.

We quickly started networking to learn how to fight cancer, and we received a lot of suggestions and information. In the six weeks before the radiation treatment commenced, we acted right away. I still have this handwritten letter I wrote her on three 14-inch yellow legalsize pages. I won't write out the names of the professionals or other advocates in the cancer fighting industry that I had written. I'll just say what they do. Also, I believe in them, even today, as much as I believe in the medical doctors. This is the letter:

> "Our game plan to good health"
>
> I decided to write you as opposed to talking to you because I realize during this crisis how you do

not listen to me, or to maybe anybody else outside of professional help, but maybe Lynn. That's why I really miss her now because if she were here maybe I could get her to give you some of my ideas.

You will actually cut me off if I say some truth that you don't want to hear or face. I've heard, "I had one daddy," fifty million times. Yet when you tell me what the family therapist said, or the Chinese doctor, the Japanese visualist, and even the hands-on therapist, many are the things that I have observed and tried to say all along.

Answer me this, "Why is everybody so nice?" family therapist, medical doctor, visualist, hands-on, and Chinese doctor.

Answer: They are in the business of being nice and are paid to be so.

For the first time since I've known you, you've allowed your body to rest. You have taken steps to relieve your mind of stress. You have taken steps to give fuel to your body to strengthen it and allow the power of the mind and body to help heal you. You have taken that nasty tea like a real trooper. I didn't think you could do it. You're a person that frowns at the aftertaste of a diet drink. You took a lot of pills in the last month. When I count them up starting with the blood pressure pills, then C, E, and Carotene, Chinese pills for the immune system, and the tea, I have to say that you've done an excellent job before the doctors started their treatment of radiation. It took them close to six weeks of tests to get you started on treatment. So you have done a good job of filling in the gaps with alternative treatments while they were testing. (I forgot shark cartilage pills, figs, almonds, asparagus, no red meat, that brown rice, and the Ensure.)

OK, now that the radiation has started we have

got to give you a break from taking too many things at this point.

I believe the radiation will work. The tests say there are traces of cancer in the bones, and radiation is supposed to be good on that; it's in the book on that bone material that I picked up. You don't have the major symptoms of swelling in the bones, vomiting, etc. So it is my guess that the radiation will work after two more good weeks of treatment.

Meanwhile let's drop the antioxidants, shark cartilage, and Chinese pills for now. We can pick them up later. That seems to be too much to take. Let them finish the radiation series, and we will do this:

(1) You can decide if you want to continue the tea for the next three weeks or start again after the radiation.

(2) A must: you must drink a *large* can of Ensure a day. This will give your body the nutrition it needs and the calories.

This tastes better than the tea, doesn't it?

(3) Eat any other food that you can. Eat whether you like it or want it. Think of it as taking medicine for the body.

(4) Meditation: keep it up. Rest and meditation would be what you would be doing if you were in a hospital. The church, visualist, hands-on, and family therapist.

a. Keep going to church: Sundays, Thursdays, and any other Bible readings.

b. Listen to more healing tapes.

c. Keep the family therapist.

d. Halt visualist and hands-on therapy during radiation. You might want to go to see them, but do you *need* to see them?

> I think it's more want than need at this time. You should know how to meditate and do the breathing exercises on your own by now. You're well acquainted with their theories. Now it is up to you to practice them on your own. We can't be under the stress of too many trips to the North Side four or five times a week while you are in pain. You know what to do. Just do it. Rest and meditate; it's a thing people have to do on their own. Break the cycle of having to be in the presence of these professionals. It's like being saved.
>
> The preacher can't do it for you. You must do it alone.
>
> Spend the next four weeks off, "on the go." You always seem to want to be on the go. Halt, relax, read, look at TV, listen to music, stop pushing your body. You know you have a problem with staying home. Relax, be waited on, be selfish, worry about yourself only. You can't be in the position to help Crystal if you are not around."

We talked for a good while after she read the letter.

Everything in these sad and desperate times was happening at a dizzying pace, and the professionals we were seeing were spread out to the far corners of Chicago. Cynthia had told me that her leg was hurting her more and more in the first week before she mentioned it to her doctor. I told her that she had to mention it and she did. I also emphasized that it was normal for her to be afraid. She didn't have to try to be extremely brave in front of me and everybody else. I told her to remember even Christ himself cried out on the cross, "Father, why hast thou forsaken me?"

I went on to say that I wasn't saying that Christ was afraid, but maybe even He was exasperated from suffering and the human death experience.

I always felt sort of strange when I quoted something from the Bible or related something to Biblical experiences. I was wondering whether she was thinking, "Bob, you don't even attend church on a regular basis."

But I had been raised in the church, and in America there's a Christian culture that extends beyond attending church. It's almost impossible to grow up in the African-American community (relating to your extended family, elderly people, Christians in general) and not be steeped in the Bible stories and quotations of scripture.

Radiation treatments had started in April. Jason, who was very close to his mother, had a very difficult time concentrating on his studies. He was due to graduate from law school in May, and there was no way Cynthia was going to miss graduation. She skipped a couple of radiation treatments so she wouldn't be too tired to attend. We stayed in a hotel on campus which was within walking distance of the graduation hall. Cyn couldn't move around, but I walked all over the campus and Jason was glad his mother was able to be there.

The radiation treatments didn't seem too physically deteriorating on Cynthia, but it did tire her out. We both hoped and believed the treatments on her leg would end the pain, but they didn't. When that became obvious, we decided to visit an Asian acupuncturist. We did that for a while, but acupuncture didn't stop the pain either. The pills prescribed by the doctor were progressively stronger, but nothing really worked well until she started on M. S. Contin and Roxanal. Cyn wouldn't take more of any of the pills than what the prescription said. The pain caused some incredible nights that I can't get out of my head. When she was moaning in pain, I thought she should have taken more pills, but she had this idea that she didn't want to get addicted to pain pills. My thinking was that I would do anything to stop the pain and worry about addiction later.

In June Cyn could still walk and breathe without a concentrator. Two of her best friends she worked with and often went to lunch with at Ameritech took her out for a weekend of relaxation. Vicky Williams, Hazel Taylor, and Cyn also sat together at church. They got reservations and a suite in a hotel in Downers Grove, Illinois in early June. I thought it was very nice of them, and it was definitely something that Cyn could use. And maybe it was a break that I needed too. I always got out of the way of Cyn and her girlfriends because she enjoyed hanging with the girls like I enjoyed hanging with my buddies.

I asked Vicky to write out the events of that weekend for me. She had talked about it with me before, but I believe that things come back to a person more detailed when it is written down.

June 1993 was the last month that Cyn could walk with ease and breathe without the help of oxygen tanks. She was now in chemotherapy, and there was no good news coming forth. She had an appointment for a second opinion at the Mayo Clinic, but she had become too sick to keep it. I called Cyn at Northwestern Hospital on my last day of school in late June. She was in for chemo. She said that they had finally found the primary tumor. And then she said, "Baby, we need a miracle."

Girlfriend

Vicky's Tale: Three Short Days

DAY ONE

It was Friday, June 4th, 1993. There were three of us looking forward to a getaway weekend. Cindy, Hazel, and I. This getaway was Cindy's idea. It came together when a friend of hers wanted to have a prayer breakfast and invited several other ladies to get together and pray for her. Although Cindy knew that she meant well, it upset her. She didn't want to be on display, so to speak. When she called me and told me how she felt about this, I just asked her to tell me what did she want. Whatever she wanted was what I would do. She said she wanted to go away for a weekend. Just the three of us. I thought that was a great idea. We both knew without saying that we wouldn't go too far from home, but far away enough to make it seem like a vacation. I called Hazel. I made the plans, the reservations, everything. It was supposed to be a flawless weekend. So many little things went awry for each of us on the day we were to leave that I would have stayed home if it had been for any other reason than to help make Cindy happy.

I had reserved a rental car with avis, but when I got there to pick up the car, the authorization hadn't gone through for the weekend package I wanted. We had reservations at the Marriott in Downers Grove but no way to get there. That's when Cindy's son Jason offered to drive us. We were heading west to pick up Hazel. It was pouring rain and the traffic was a bear because the Bulls were hot in the finals and there was a game that night. I'm a Bulls fan, and neither Cindy nor Hazel was. (I feel bad now for wanting to see the game that night.)

When we finally arrived at the hotel, I got out and went in. I was met at the front door by the concierge. Because I had preregistered, the keys were waiting at the front door. I returned to the car to get my buddies so quickly the first thing Cindy said was, "What's wrong now?"

I said, "Nothing," and flashed the keys. Well, we were there. Way out in Downers Grove. With no way back home unless we called for someone to come and get us. A very nice bellhop helped us to our suite. In keeping with the glitches of the day, the accommodations in the suite were not what I had requested. So what else could go wrong? The bellhop called to the front desk to get us a better suite. I looked at Cindy and I could see she was getting very tired. I took her purse and coat from her and sat her down on the gurney with our bags. I'm a real mother hen sometimes. We finally got into our suite and began unpacking.

After a short while, we were talking and for a while it seemed like none of us had any problems. We were just "the girlfriends" having fun. Cindy offered to take the sofa in the living room because she said she coughed so badly at night. I told her I wouldn't have it; for she and Hazel were to take to the bedroom, Cindy was to be as comfortable as possible. We ordered room service. I caught a little of the game on TV. We were really wiped out. We bedded down rather early. We dozed off, I think. I heard Cindy coughing in the next room. I slid quietly from the sofa bed and got down on my knees to pray. I cried silently and prayed. She coughed. I cried… I prayed… she coughed. Then I heard angels singing. I thought I was imagining the singing so I prayed harder. I still heard music and singing. Then I realized Hazel had awakened too. She was softly playing gospel tapes to try to help Cindy relax. It was obvious that we were all awake in the wee hours with only one prayer request on our minds. A prayer for a miracle, a healing.

We all got together in the living room of our suite and prayed out loud. We held each other, cried, prayed, and welcomed the presence of Jesus' Holy Spirit into our midst. And…

He showed up! "Where two or three are gathered together in my name there I am in the midst of them." Matt. 18:20

DAY TWO

Now is it early Saturday or very late Friday. Either way we watched the sun come up. Cindy didn't feel like going down for breakfast, even though it was included in our weekend package. Hazel and I dressed and went for breakfast while Cindy rested. We brought Cindy some juice and light breakfast food to go with her Ensure. Hazel convinced Cindy to get up and get dressed to go outside and get some fresh air. We walked among the garden flowers. I had remembered to bring a camera. We took pictures and managed to clown around a bit. Hazel was really the balancing force. She had lost both parents to this horrible disease and knew more about it than I did. I was just trying to be strong in a helpless kind of way. The rest of the day was spent back in our room bonding with each other even more.

Later on we ordered dinner via room service. The bathroom had a double entrance, one door faced the living room and the other door, of course, was off the bedroom. After dinner Cindy went to the bathroom to shampoo her hair. She still had a lot of hair.

I was more or less watching over her than watching her that weekend. I was sitting on the couch in the living room watching her leaning over the bathroom sink trying to rinse her hair when I saw that she was crying. I didn't tell Hazel,

I just got up and walked through the bedroom and into the bathroom from the side entrance. I started rinsing her hair for her and said "I'll bet the two of us together can get this done faster than just one of us alone." We both shed more tears as we rinsed her beautiful head of hair. I hugged her as I towel dried it. Guess what? She even let me comb it!

Well, as our second day was ending it was time to start trying to figure out how we were going to get to church in the morning. I had an idea. I called a limousine service and arranged for us to get to church in style.

DAY THREE

We had an early morning prayer and got ready for church. Our limo was waiting. Cindy was smiling. The mission was accomplished. What had started out as a real bummer had turned into a blessed event. Cindy sat in the limo facing Hazel and me. She looked regal. We rode in style down the highway and on to church. I remember Cindy saying "Vic, you sure know how to live!" It was June 6, 1993. I was sure she would get better. That was 198 days before she left us.

I have included a poem by Hazel, who was the other good friend on that three-day trip. Hazel and her husband, Gary, are a very talented couple; Gary is an artist and Hazel is a poet. Cyn and I had purchased some of his great works. I won't be able to reproduce the little drawings of flowers Hazel had between the verses of her poem. The blossoms were painted red, and the stems were green. It put a smile on Cyn's face, even though at that time she had gone into the stage where she didn't want to see anybody.

God sends so many people
    into our lives —
Some bring us smiles,
    some bring us tears —
Some bring us
    unexplainable joy —
While others bring us
    fears
Some bring us truths
    we cannot bear —
Some bring us lies
    that are filled with pain —
But, yet and still,
    from all of these —
There's something to be
    gained.
With You, He sent
    that special smile —
Showing others that YOU
    really care —
YOUR greeting —
    "HOW YA' DO'N SWEETHEART" —
And YOUR willingness
    to share.
The words escape me
    when we talk —
But I feel the need to let
    YOU know —
I'm glad GOD put YOU
    in my life —
Allowing Me to LOVE YOU so!

– HAZEL M. TAYLOR
JULY 29, 1993

Loathe to Leave

A time of grave illness abounds in sadness. It is full of days and nights that you would graciously forget, if you could. But this time also abounds in feelings of intense love. For one, it's the last great act of giving and sharing. It's the reality of we'll always be together, I'll always love you, and "till death do us part." This is one night and one day of loving, giving, and sharing that stays in my head.

One night in the first days of Cynthia's illness, for the first time, she allowed herself to wallow in self-pity out loud. She wasn't hysterical, but softly crying and talking about fighting cancer and the possibility of dying. She spoke of things like not wanting to lose her hair during radiation, and leaving her kids. I was sitting on the sofa, and she was sitting on my lap. I had my arms around her trying to console her, and she told me, "I don't want you to give pleasure to anybody else."

I said, "Sweetheart, that's the last thing you should be thinking about right now. You know can't any woman ever take your place."

After saying a few more things she went to sleep with her head on my chest. She understandably hadn't slept well the last couple of nights. So I sat there holding her, and she slept for a little over an hour. We were going to a prayer meeting at church that night; I knew she didn't want to miss it, so I woke her up to either go, or get in the bed. She wanted to go and we did.

I thought a lot about what she had said to me, about me going on and finding a life with another woman. I thought it was just natural for someone in love to do, but it was so sad to me then, and it's very sad to me now. It is a part of my strong feelings of how life was so unfair to her. Taking away her life brutally, taking her away from her kids, and giving her lover, her husband, to another woman by default. I guess, thinking about your mate going on without you is normal for one deeply in love. I know that if I were in the same position, it would have been a part of my thinking, a part of my jealous feelings of possessiveness. But she didn't have time to dwell on that. If she dwelled on anything, it was about not wanting to leave her children. To me, she said on one occasion, "You're going to find somebody else." She said it so casually that it really bothered me. How could she think I could just go on rather easily? I was thinking,

"After all of these years, and all of the ways I have tried to tell her the depths of my love and my need for her, I've still fallen short. I can't just find somebody else. I don't want anybody else. I needed her to stay here with me."

But I couldn't bring a subject like that back up; I couldn't belabor a point about how I would be after she was gone. That would have been completely self-serving. She was fighting for her life, and we needed to just concentrate on that. Besides, I think it was just sort of a test. She just wanted to hear me say again how much I loved her, how much I would miss her, and knowing how sweet and caring she was, I believe it was her way of releasing me to try and be happy again.

All during her illness, I had to be very tactful in my language, and mostly respond to questions and issues that she brought up. She was too sharp mentally for me to say things in a round about way, especially, since we had always been straightforward. She left me an opening one day when talking about her children, and I distinctly remember assuring her that I would always look out for her babies if they let me.

By now she couldn't walk. She was in a wheelchair. The long cord from the oxygen concentrator machine strapped around her face and was in her nose. She wore a very pretty scarf on her head for no other reason than fading vanity, because there was nobody in the house but us. Though her hair was gone, eyebrows frizzled, and her eyes had a slightly sunken look, she was my baby, the quintessential female to me... still the most beautiful and exciting woman in the world.

She asked me to push her to the front door so she could look out. I told her my concerns about it being too cool for a person in a robe. Her voice was clear and stern; she wanted to sit a while. She just wanted to sit and look at the outdoors. I did what she asked and left the room not knowing whether she wanted to pray, cry, or merely have quiet time alone. She called in just a few minutes, saying in her quiet and always polite way, "Bobby, I'm ready."

Her face was impassive, and her eyes dry when I came into the room. I pulled the chair and closed the door. She said, "Put me back in the bed."

I wanted desperately for her to share her thoughts with me, but I could see she wasn't going to say anything. I lifted her out of the chair to the side of the bed, pushed the chair out the way, fluffed the pillows, swung both legs around off the floor, then pulled her up on the pillows with both of my arms under hers. I asked if she wanted any mineral ice on her left leg, which hurt all the time. She said yes. When I finished rubbing it on, I wrapped one heating pad around her leg and placed the other at the base of her back.

When she was comfortable, I sat on the side of the bed trying to get her to share her thoughts. I said, "You had a far-away look in your eyes."

She didn't respond. I continued, "Looking over my vast estate, huh?"

I should have outright asked her to share her thoughts

with me, but I didn't want to push anything. I was always afraid that I was going to say the wrong thing, something that would precipitate a flood of tears, a swing of her mood into a wave of self-pity. It was a thing I would do sometimes as I was riding around in my car. I was always thinking about my sweet, sweet baby in pain, and of her being gravely ill.

Because it was overcast and gray I said, "It's not a very pretty day, huh?

She disagreed and was barely audible saying, "It was nice."

I said, "You wanna rest? …You wanna talk?

She shook her head saying no, and I took it to mean no to talking. I said, "OK, Babe, call me if you need me."

When I was in my room thinking about the look on her face, what it said, what she didn't say, some of what she was thinking came to me. She had asked me before to put a chair out on the front porch so she could sit and think a while. Some nights we would sit on the front steps for a short while, but for the most part this was not our pattern. The look on her face made one thing perfectly clear — every day the Lord has made is a good day. A day to give thanks and praise. Today was gray, but it would soon change to sunshine; if not tomorrow, the next day or week. The seasons will also change because it's all a part of a grand design. She didn't want to leave her children or me, and also not this pretty place. Like all of us, she didn't want to leave the Earth. Is this not Eden, physically? Heaven must really be a grand-looking place for the Lord to top his creation here. And this is another reason we loathe to leave in spite of believing that we're going to Heaven, in spite of the promise of everlasting life in a place we've never been.

Eartharina

Loathe to leave
this beautiful place
landscaped by
the hand of Grace.

mountains
valleys
windswept plains
water lily ponds
gentle falling rains.

loathe to leave
a sunshiny day
snow storms
rain forests
ocean spray,

meadows of stallions
autumn leaves
redwoods
palms
cottonwood trees.

loathe to leave
fields of maize
hot
snowy
foggy
overcast days,

coral reefs
butterflies
creatures
of the woods
the sea and the skies.

loathe to leave
a starlit skyline
autumn
winter
spring
summertime,

a sun setting
in an orange
and purple sky,

this must be Eden
don't want
to say goodbye.

save me Jesus
I don't want to die.

The Last Summer

In the spring Cynthia left work on a medical leave. She was already sleeping in the room across from our bedroom; the rooms were about eight feet apart. She stayed up late reading and looking at television, so she needed a room of her own. It was my son's room before he left and went south to go to school. When Cyn went in for chemo one time, Jason helped me paint the room white, change things around, and I got some different curtains. The rooms were so close together, she could speak to me in her normal voice and I would hear her in the next room.

Cyn would never miss church while she could still walk. At the beginning of her illness, I started attending church with her. But I only attended a few times. I felt a little hypocritical, but that was not the main reason I wasn't there with her for as long as she could attend. I thought she needed to be with her spiritual friends in a normal situation without my presence. I knew she drew strength from them, and I wanted her to be able to act normally as she did when I was not around. I wanted her to cry if she wanted, to stay for any special prayers, or to just talk to her friends. It was normal for me not to be there, and I wanted to try to maintain normalcy.

One night during an intercessory prayer meeting, the ladies gathered around her for that hard praying they could really do at Apostolic. They knew she was sick, and they probably prayed even harder. I sat a few rows back observing and praying on my own. Their voices got real loud; they were touching and hugging. Soon, Cyn fell back, and they gently laid her on the floor. There were a couple of other people lying on the floor also. I remembered something like this from television, but I had never seen it in person. I moved closer and sat in the front row. I didn't know any of the women but Edna Thompson, a fellow teacher. Edna had given Cyn a book on healing. She told me not to worry; everything would be all right. Cyn lay on the floor for maybe 20 minutes. I just sat there watching her and watching the little kids that were walking around her, moving back and forth as though they were used to this. When she opened her eyes they lifted her up and they talked and hugged. On the way home she told me, "Bobby, I hope you weren't afraid."

I said I had been a little apprehensive, but I could tell by the reaction that it must have been normal and expected for this type of meeting. Then Cyn asked me had anybody touched her while she was on the floor. She said she felt as though hands were pressing on her. I told her no, and I was watching her all of the time. She asked, "Do you think I was touched by the hand of God?"

I said, "You weren't touched by anybody else while you were on the floor."

I knew that even with my crash course in praying and spirituality I was out of my league. My best bet was to do what I've always done: get out of the way. Let her be with the church friends she has always been with, but go along with her if she asked. She didn't ask, so I assumed I was right.

I was very glad for so many reasons when the school year ended in June, 1993. It was the hardest year of my teaching career. Now, for at least 10 weeks, I could devote myself full-time to taking care of Cynthia, and also help out with Crystal. Jason was home from law school now. He would be a really big help for me and his mother. He didn't hesitate; his sense of duty to his mother and sister was simply outstanding.

It was sometime in the middle of June that Cyn began taking oxygen. At first I thought she needed something to help her breathe better without it being a dire need. It was not like one day she couldn't breathe and we rushed her to the emergency room to get oxygen. The severity of the need was between her and her doctor. I could easily see the need for the wheelchair, because she obviously had trouble walking. In the weeks before school was out, I would take Cyn over to her mother's apartment while I was at work, sometimes just to stay and visit. We rented a second oxygen concentrator machine to stay at her mother's apartment. We used the tanks mainly to go to and from the doctor's office and to the hospital.

I had always been a light sleeper, but throughout her illness I became an even lighter sleeper. She had instructions to call me absolutely every time she needed me. This was for anytime of night, no matter how many times it had to be. But I would always get up to check on her anyway. I wanted to make sure the oxygen cord was in her nose. Sometimes it came out while she was sleeping, so I was very vigilant.

It seemed like Cyn being in the wheelchair just naturally happened. She could hardly walk at all, and she needed it to go to the bathroom. I would help her into the chair, push her into the bathroom, and wait until she called me. Early in the summer I could still leave her in the house while I made a quick trip to the store. She could be in bed, or sitting in the wheelchair in the living room. I always preferred to wait until Jason came over before I left the house. Cyn's mother was in her eighties, and although she wanted to help there was really not much she could do. Cyn needed lift-and-push help. Crystal would come over every once in a while, but not too much because Cyn wanted it that way. She didn't believe Crystal was strong enough to deal with what was going on.

When Cyn first started going to the hospital for chemo or getting fluid drained from her lungs, she asked me to pick her up a new robe and sleeping gown. It was something I hadn't done before, but I did pick out some pretty ones. She wrote a special note to me, which made me feel really gratified. I was back picking out things for my lady. She liked how we had painted the room and had all of the medicine and everything in order and easily accessible.

There were several church members who came by for prayer sessions. I wouldn't be in the room, but I would always close my eyes and listen. I really admired the way they could pray, and it was very comforting to Cyn. A friend of Cyn's, Pat Hayes, brought her minister by to pray one day also. Cyn would talk on the telephone a lot at first, but there soon came a time when there were just too many calls. I had to monitor the length of the calls because they tired her out. There also came a time when she simply didn't want to talk to anybody. Everybody understood when I told them.

During the time when Cyn could still walk, a lot of our optimism for her getting well would come from talking to cancer survivors and patients she would meet at the doctor's office. She would also attend support group meetings. Many survivors had been ill for five years or more, and some had gone into remission. One survivor, Nola, was very inspirational for Cynthia. I never met her, but she was the very nice lady who let Cyn wear a Catholic medal that she had worn. As I can recall, when Nola found out she had cancer, she started wearing the medal. One day a white dove appeared in a tree near her home. The dove remained in the tree for the whole day. When she went back to the doctor for a checkup there was no trace of the cancer. Cyn met Nola through a mutual friend, Sonia, and Nola was gracious enough to send the medal in the hope that it would do the same miracle for Cyn. I know they talked back and forth for a few months before Cyn sent her the medal back because Nola's cancer had returned. But while Cyn had the medal, we were looking for a miracle, and we were looking for a dove. We knew that a dove is one of the symbols for the Holy Spirit.

After Cyn's death, her mother told me that on one of her visits Cyn asked her, "Mama, can't you see that I'm dying?"

Her Mother replied, "Baby, don't say that. You don't know that."

But Cyn continued with, "Mama, I wont be here with you much longer." And they hugged and cried together.

Cyn and I never discussed dying. She asked me on one of my visits to her room at Northwestern Hospital, "Why are you looking so sad?"

I replied, "I just can't be my old happy self while you're sick and going through pain. I'm sorry, but I can't play those games some books say I should play. I'm praying all the time. I have faith in God that everything is going to be all right, but I can't be my old self. We were on our honeymoon, right? But I'll try much harder baby, if it would help you to feel better."

She said she understood. Cyn knew I wasn't the deceptive type.

She always said that I couldn't keep a secret, and everything showed on my face. Anyway, it was just hugging and praying time.

It was so unusual not to have any disagreements, or not to fuss about this or that. I was used to her getting a little miffed at me about some small matter from time to time. And it did happen one day while she was sick. She always said that I was the type that was not picky about eating, and she was. So I knew we were going to have some disagreements over me trying to push her to eat disagreeable-tasting food, those medicinal types of foods. I was always on some liquid diet with protein drinks, diet sodas, and all, but she hated that sort of eating. She loved fancy foods and different types of cuisines. She and Lynn had tried unsuccessfully to get me to eat escargots one time. It was just set in my mind that massive dosages of foods and vitamins that were supposed to fight cancer were in order for Cyn to take. I figured they just might work. I wanted her to take and eat as many of the vitamins and foods as I could. She sensed I was disappointed and thought that I was even mad at her because she couldn't. She had gotten out of bed and called me up from my word processor in the basement. She walked with a limp and had one arm on the wall helping to hold herself up. I was up the steps fast. I met her in the living room. She asked, "You've been down there a long time. Are you mad at me?"

I was grabbing her around the waist to walk her back to the bedroom. I said, "Mad at you? What made you think that?"

She replied, "Babe, I'm doing the best I can. I can't eat as much of this stuff as you can."

It was said so sincerely, and she looked so helpless that thinking about it has moistened my eyes several times since. I have to fight back tears when I think about it today. I told her, "No, I'm not mad at you. I know you're trying your best. But you know I'm going to have to push you a little."

I had her back in bed in no time. I was sitting on the side of the bed and got me some sugah before adding, "No, I'm going to have to push you a lot. But I could never be mad at you. You're fighting hard, and you're very brave. You know I got to make sure my baby is around. I don't wanna be the saddest man in the world."

Then I made a mistake. I never wanted to say anything negative, something about dying, but I said something, and I thought right away that it was wrong. "Remember Cyn, I'll hold you to your word. You said you'll never leave me."

I wanted to take it back right away. It was so stupid. It was like saying that she had made herself sick. Thankfully, she just squeezed me. I felt like crying, but we didn't cry. We just held each other without saying anything. Then I said, "I just hope I'm doing the right things."

And she said, "You are, Baby… I know you're trying hard, too, and you're my rock."

It was the most loving thing she could have said to me. It was even better than saying, "I love you," again. I was doing everything I could to make her as comfortable as possible — buying things for her and waiting on her hand and foot. She knew to wake me up, no matter what the time was, if she needed me to take her to the washroom, pull her up in the bed, or even just to pray with her. Still, I felt I was really doing nothing. She was the brave one, the one in pain and going through the mind games of being terminally ill. All along I thought she was playing the mind game much better than I was. I was sort of in awe of the fact that she was not mentally falling apart right in front of my face. Her nature was to be overly sentimental about bad things happening to members of her family and people that she loved. And here she was… strong-willed with a strong faith that things were going to turn out all right.

I'm thinking specifically about one night in late spring, maybe four months after the diagnosis of her illness. It was around 11:30, and I was in my room in bed because I had to go to work in the morning. It was before she had to use oxygen or a wheelchair. But as I have stated, since she stayed up late reading and watching television, she slept in the other room across from me. She came into the room and got into what was normally our bed and our room. She snuggled up to me saying, "How long has it been since we made love?"

I said, "I don't remember. It ain't been on my mind for a long time."

She replied, "Mine either… until tonight."

I was quick, "Wait a minute. You don't have to do this for me."

She said, "It's the first time I have felt like doing it for months."

I was more than just reluctant, I was really nervous about it. She was very thin, and the radiation treatments on her leg and hip had left dark spots like burns. I didn't know whether it would hurt her or not. I wanted to reassure her that I was OK with things as they were.

"Really sweet, I'm OK. Your wifely duty right now is to get well."

But hugging and snuggling closer she said, "Bob, it's all right; I want to for the first time in months. I'm going to beat this thing anyway."

She was talking about beating cancer, and her mood was more upbeat than I had seen it in months, so how could I resist? She was very loving, but very thin. So thin that I could feel her rib cage against me. Also somehow, I just knew it was the last time we would make love. I felt as though the lovemaking was more for me. She was just sweet that way.

She lay with me a little while and gave me a lot of wet kisses before going back into her bed across the hall. In about three minutes, she called out saying, "Baby, we forgot to pray. I want you to start off tonight. Don't get out of the bed. I can hear you from here."

I said, "OK... we'll say the Lord's Prayer together."

And we lay in our beds and recited the Lord's Prayer in a duet as we always did. Then she said, "Good night, Babe, sleep tight."

In about two minutes, I got out of my bed and went into her room. I got on my knees and held one of her hands.

"Cyn, I got to get a little more personal with the Lord than reciting the Lord's Prayer. I got to talk to Him personally, to let him know how much I need my bride around."

So I prayed first, and she came right in praying as I finished. It was our standard practice. When we had finished, I showered her with wet kisses and left the room.

The sad thoughts would not leave my mind. She was so innocent but still attacked by this dreadful disease. And lying alone in the dark, the full force of the idea of being without her hit me. Our house had always been a place of happiness. When I closed and locked the front door, we were safe from harm. Magic and love were all around. Now, like a fog, sadness slithered through that space under our door that only something vapor-like could pass under. It headed straight to my room and lay heavily in the air.

Our rooms were so close we could hear each other's loud breathing. So I had to be careful not to make any noise accidentally hitting things. When I became really sad, my eyes would moisten. But I had replaced crying with striking out at something. When a person cries during times like these, it's not for himself. It's that sadness you feel for what your loved one is going through. When they're gone, then you cry for yourself.

On that night, I was in a rage of anger and extreme sadness. It made me want to walk around hard in circles, cussing, and slamming things down. Something about the night had just told me that we would never be normal again. We had been on the cancer battlefield for about four months, and the fighting had consumed our concentration. One sweet gesture changed everything. Suddenly, it was not hugs for comforting. Not loving, but non-passionate type kisses on the jaw. That night we were lovers again, and that return to normalcy and hearing Cyn's optimism against fading odds had overwhelmed me. It was like a beginning and an end happening at the same time.

I didn't want to get out of the bed and walk around because she would hear me. I wanted to, but I couldn't just get up and go for a walk around the block. This had been a loving and pleasant night for both of us; I wanted it to remain that way. I just had to find a way to deal with my agony while staying in bed. I put my head under the pillow and started hitting my fist on the bed. I kept thinking about Cyn. How much I loved her, needed her in my life, and how hard she was trying. I kept thinking, "My poor baby! She's trying so hard. Wanting to live and not leave her children. Wanting to be a wife and just a woman again." I tried, but I couldn't will myself out of that fit of anger and thinking over and over, "It ain't fair! ...my poor baby!"

And I stayed in that fit of hitting the mattress with my fist and praying, "God please save her..." until I fell off to sleep.

I was really prepared to do what we were doing for years to come. I thought maybe she would die from cancer, but we had years. If the doctors could have found a way to stop her pain, I was going to find a way to make life worth living for her.

I was going to love her, and wait on her, I was going to make her smile again. And we would both thank God just for being alive. It wasn't to be, but Cyn, Jason, and I would give it our best shot.

Mammy

I'm always reaching out for things that will help pull me through these days, and the voices of great preachers are always comforting. Along with the moving voice of Cyn's and my pastor, Bishop Brazier, I thought about one of my heroes from African-American history. I wanted to read and imagine hearing the great voice of James Weldon Johnson. So I read again from his book, *God's Trombones*.

This is a book of seven sermons by this brave, black leader. He looked so white he was able to attend a southern lynching and write about it. He was a poet, activist, college professor, and preacher. Reading his book helped me in my grieving. I think of Cynthia's son, daughter, and myself when reading the moving poem, "Go Down Death — A Funeral Sermon"

This is the first verse:

> Weep not, Weep not,
> She is not dead;
> she's resting in the bosom of Jesus.
> Heart-broken husband — weep no more;
> Grief-stricken son — weep no more;
> Left-lonesome daughter — weep no more;
> She's only just gone home.

Even though he was not in the regular literature text books used in high school in those "Jim Crow" days, our black teachers brought him and other black poets into the classroom. They were taught right along with Shakespeare and Poe. This verse is near the end of another great poem by James Weldon Johnson; it's also in *God's Trombones.* When I was in grade and high school, there were contests between students to recite and act out *The Creation.*

> This Great God
> Like a mammy bending over her baby
> Kneeled down in the dust
> Toiling over a lump of clay
> Till he shaped it in his own image.

This line, "Like a mammy bending over her baby," was the main reason I bought myself another copy of the book. It was a line that came to mind one night during Cynthia's illness, and it stayed in my head while I was taking care of Cyn in her worst days. It moved me to name this chapter, Mammy.

In any relationship with a woman, a man plays several roles. I was a friend, lover, protector, soulmate, husband, and according to Cynthia, a rock. During the worst weeks of her illness, I had to go a step further than those roles, which were fun and easy to play. They're roles most guys can perform all right with because they're gender roles. A man goes through gender training all of his life. I had been lucky throughout my life in that I had never lived with anyone that was ill over a period of time and needed special care. Now I had to take care of and help make critical decisions for a loved one with a dreaded and possibly terminal disease.

Living alone with your mate is great when there's no illness involved, but when there is, it's really helpful psychologically and physically to have a big family around. In James Weldon Johnson's *The Creation*, he personified God "Like a mammy bending over her baby." This is an extremely powerful image to me. It's the essence of the Earth Mother, and a natural portrait of one of the most maligned personages in African-American history. She's a heroine unheralded and a revolutionist defamed. It was she that held the slave family together; she that was forced to be a wet nurse to her enemy's children. She was forced to help raise the child that perhaps one day would order the beatings and even death of her own child. But while she helped raise the master's son with one hand, she raised an insurrectionist with the other. Also, maybe the worst, I don't know, she was denied the image of grace, svelteness, beauty, and femininity of other women. But obviously she must have been desirable and beautiful. Without a doubt, she was the greatest victim of miscegenation.

The time had come in my long love affair with Cynthia when she needed more of me than the gender roles I had been taught to play. She needed more than a lover or leading man. Like many other men who had been in my position, and those who are presently in the same situation, I had to play a new role. I thought about it one night when I was bending over Cynthia, "Like a mammy bending over her baby."

Cyn had asked me about why I was looking so sad, and I had forced myself to act in a more chipper, if not a cheerful manner. So after putting her back in bed and pulling her up on the pillows so she could be comfortable, I said, "Well, sweet thang. I'm gonna take care of you, and it won't be like the proverbial daddy you always accused me of playing."

There was a joking joviality when I continued with, "Baby… um gonna be yo mammy."

Cyn's condition was deteriorating. I didn't see the change coming clearly, but all of a sudden in the last weeks of her illness, it was just there. She needed a different type of help because before I knew it, there were two Cindys. One I had known and had loved for the last 18 years, even though at this time she was not exactly herself. No longer the glamorous, sassy, independent woman she had always been, but still a fighter with a strong faith and will. The new Cindy's mind was strong, but she was helpless and dependent, very much like a baby. Her voice, which was always a rich, polished, oval sound had changed. All of a sudden, it was a light, high-pitched whisper. She sounded just like a little girl. I think it was from swollen lymph glands in her neck that were pressing against her vocal cords. I'm guessing, I was not sure. But like Cindy as her old self, my new Cindy's speech was very mannered and polite. Always gently asking something and afterwards saying a sweet "Thank you," as if she needed to thank me.

I carried her to the bathtub; it wasn't easy, but the warm water helped her leg. She picked up washing off with these plastic tubs from the hospital, and she liked doing that frequently. I would wash her back and dry her off. I always made sure that she was smelling nice, and that the room was clean and smelled good. I had observed how the nurses would do things, how they used sheets to pull her up in the bed, and I copied their method.

Cyn would always tell me when she wanted to go to the bathroom. I pushed the wheelchair into the bathroom and closed the door. Using her arms on the cabinet, she could manage on her own for the first few months. Soon that became difficult for her. When she was in Northwestern Hospital, I noticed the nurse had stopped using the bedpans, but had this little portable toilet by the bed. I bought one for her room at home, but before that I had to use strong conversation to get things straight about matters of vanity.

"Cyn, I know what vanity is, and I know what needs to be done. I know you would prefer your mama to help you, but she's not here; she couldn't do the job anyway. I only want to have to say this once. I'm going to do what's necessary to do. If you're constipated, I can give an enema like the nurse can. This is no time to be vain or ashamed. You're going to be as clean and smelling good as you've always been. If the time comes when we need to hire a part-time nurse, we can do that too."

In spite of my overall down mood, I had learned to be my jivey self, and I continued, "But, Babe… you got me all the time. And I'm going to do for you what I know you would do for me. That's just the way it's gonna be. Are we absolutely clear on that? …OK good."

I bought all sorts of stuff for her comfort and functional use. But the one thing I really could have used at home was one of those electric adjustable beds. Sometimes I would sleep in her bed until she was asleep. Then I would slide out and go to my bed for the rest of the night. It reminded me of sleeping with my boy when he was an infant. I would fall asleep, and then feel this soft nudging for me to wake up. And when I turned and we looked into each other's eyes, she would say in that light sweet voice, "I wanna go to the bathroom."

And I don't know exactly why, but I even started talking softer like I was talking to a toddler, "All right, Sweetheart; anything you say."

A lot of the times she wanted to sit in the wheelchair in the living room. While I moved her in and out and tucked her back into the bed, she would always pat me on the face. And always before I would go to the other room, I had to get me some sugah. Her hair was gone from radiation, but it was starting to come back; it was very fine and very soft. So I would rub her on the head and then kiss her on it. It was round, warm, and smelled real nice.

"That's some good head sugah, baby. Your hair will be back in no time. Kissing you on the head now is like doing it when you were a baby. But you are my baby, right?"

She didn't say much. I guess because I was chattering all the time, and got me some sweet sugah all the time. But her eyes would always follow me, like a precious infant's would, as I moved in and out of the room. Then I could give my stare with a half-smile. That look that said, "Baby, everything's going to be all right." But I wondered if she were thinking sometimes, "Bobby, don't you know how sick I am?"

I could never sleep really soundly, and I had the medicine schedule written down so I could wake her up when it was time. I didn't even have to set my alarm. I would get up and tiptoe to look into the room to make sure the oxygen was in her nose and everything was all right. I would look at her frail self and think to myself, "If it is your will, God, please save her."

When I would look in the room at my different Cindy sleeping, I realized I had fallen in love again. I know it was the same person, but she was so helpless and different that another type of love dominated Eros or romantic love. She was just so sweet and precious, if love was the medicine that would save her, she could have just gotten up out of that bed and gone dancing.

I can't remember being scared much during my adult life. However, these were times when I would be just plain scared. When she would visit the doctor, I wanted desperately to hear some good news. Waiting for her to tell me what progress was being made was tough. As I lay in my bed those last weeks, I was so scared that one morning I would wake up and she would be gone. So when she would call my name at night in a soft voice, and especially in a strong voice, I would be so happy. A smile would be on my face, and I would sling my legs quickly out of that bed to the floor, and I'd be in that room in no time. I placed my hand on her near-clean head, rubbing her fine, soft hair. Then it was sugah time. I'd plant my lips on her clean-smelling, warm, round head... sniffing and lingering for a few seconds. The feeling was so heavenly; she was my baby, my one and only. Then I would baby-talk whisper, "Hey, pretty girl... I'm here. Now what do you want with the love of your life?"

I hated for school to start in the fall of 1993. I just wanted to stay at home and be with her. For a teacher, normally after the summer vacation you're energized, pumped up, and anxious to meet your new crop of kids. You're hoping that all five of your classes will be nice, but you know that there's at least one headache class, and in a tough year, maybe two. Those who keep pushing the idea that school should be year round have not taught five classes for nine months in the public school system.

I thought I would have to hire a home-care nurse to look after Cynthia once school had started, but Jason wasn't about to leave his mama by finding a job in another city. He was really a big help. After a certain point, I couldn't have made it without him. We had to lift Cyn in the wheelchair to get her down my steps. Then one of us would fold the chair and place it in the trunk while the other helped Cyn into the car. This also meant coordinating our efforts with the portable oxygen tank. Jason was indispensable.

Like most people, I always wondered about the thoughts of terminally ill people. I'm still wondering. I was hoping that Cyn would share some of her thoughts with me. I believe that after a point, the fight itself with a painful disease is the consuming thought. It's just wanting the pain and discomfort to end, and to simply have a good day. I think that extreme pain might be one of nature's ways of helping a patient to let go of sweet life. Obviously, because life is no longer sweet, it has become a minute-to-minute struggle. Nobody wants to live in constant excruciating pain, and nobody wants to see it.

In the last few weeks, Cynthia's mind was clear most of the time, but the morphine did make her disoriented and talk out of her head sometimes. I was thinking that maybe I was giving her too much, so I tried to regulate it better. I read the labels carefully, called the doctors, and her reaction was somewhat normal. Some of the things she was repeating when she was disoriented were coming from the television, so I called Vicky to bring me some tapes from church. By this time Cyn did not want to talk on the telephone. She didn't want to see anybody anymore either; even those who wanted to come over to pray. So now the praying was in my hands; the man she had taught how to pray. I distinctly remember Vicky's last visit. I had sort of pushed Cyn because I knew Vicky was one of her spiritual friends, and I wanted her to keep a spiritual connection. I let Vicky in and hung up her coat. I didn't go in the room, but I could see Cyn reaching her arms up to hug her. I was very moved and very glad Vicky had come over.

Cyn would go into the hospital for a few days' stay in early December. At this time she was mostly on home-care and fading fast. Looking at how much weight she was losing and her refusing to eat hardly anything prompted me to tell my brother in November that at that rate of weight loss, I didn't think she would make it to Christmas. She slept most of the time. I was satisfied with that because that was preferable to her being in pain. The morphine was definitely effective on pain, and Jason and I made sure we had enough available for her. I thought about how so many people probably couldn't afford to buy the high-priced morphine, and I wondered if this meant that they just had to suffer that much more. I felt sorry for people I didn't even know because it all seemed so unfair.

One cold night in early December, I was in my bed sleeping and Cyn was also sleeping. About 1:00A.M. she called me in a very loud voice. It startled me because her voice was usually soft. It was a loud, panicky sounding, "Bobby!"

My feet hit the floor, and in no time I was standing over her. She said in a loud, gargled sound, "Call 911!"

Yellow fluid was bubbling out of her mouth. It was my first real panic-type situation. I said, "OK babe, but first I'm going to turn you over, so the fluid can run out better."

I pulled her up, so her face could be pointing down, and then I sort of patted her on the back like you would burp a baby. She was coughing and throwing up fluid. But it cleared up fast and she could breath all right again. I asked her did she still want me to call 911. She was still shaken by the whole thing and nodded her head yes. The 911 operator told me it would take a while, so I quickly got the phone book and called a private ambulance service. I got the quickest one to come right out.

"They're on their way, Baby."

Her eyes kept looking at me, and they had that soft, helpless look. Kissing and hugging her, I said, "It's gonna be all right, Baby. I'll be right here, but I'm going to quickly put on my clothes."

When the paramedics arrived, they talked about carrying her to the nearest hospital because it was the law, but I insisted on Northwestern. I told them I had talked to her doctor and he said to bring her there.

It was cold, but it wasn't freezing and there wasn't any snow. The street was empty of any cars or people; it was just the ambulance and us in front of our house. It was very quiet, and the red light on the top of the ambulance was spinning silently around. I felt like all the rest of the world was asleep, just going on as normal. Nobody was awake but me, these attendants, and Cyn fighting for her life. They wheeled her into the back of the ambulance and started trying to put the I.V. in her arm. Her arm was so small, they were having trouble finding her vein. I had gotten impatient; telling them to hurry and get her to the hospital, but the paramedic was patient with me. He told me to try to calm down; that this was procedure. I thought it was hurting her, even though she wasn't saying anything. They finally got it in her arm and told me not to try to stay behind them, but to meet them at the emergency room. I thought I was prepared for the end, but on my way down I kept saying, "Not now, Lord… Please not now."

Northwestern's emergency room was full, as usual, but soon we were in one of the stalls.

"Hey, girl… my baby's all right. I wanna say you scared me, but I know you're thinking that you were the one that was really scared. I told the Lord I need you to stay in my life, and he agreed."

It still took them a while to get around to her and do what they had to do before rolling her up to a room. By this time in her illness, I had mastered wearing the mask and speaking with much more confidence than I really had. I waited outside when the female intern asked me to do so. The curtain was closed a long time, so I went outside for a little fresh air. The curtain was still closed when I got back, but it opened with the intern calling my name. When I rushed over she said, "Cindy has been calling for you; apparently she can't go anywhere without you."

Cyn reached for my hand. That statement had put a smile on her face, which was something I had not seen for a long time. It brightened me up, too, and I grabbed her hand and kissed her on the jaw saying, "I can't go anywhere without her either."

She stayed in the hospital for about a week. They drained about a quart and a half of fluid off her lungs. She had to stay longer because one lung had been punctured, though with the fluid gone, she seemed more energetic than in a long time. She was so energetic that she kept pulling the oxygen out of her nose. I kept putting it back, but she was disoriented and kept pulling it out.

While she was in the hospital, Cyn's good girlfriend Carol called the house with the intention of inviting us to a Christmas party. She was really shaken when I told her about Cyn's condition; she came to the hospital the very next day. Carol always claimed that she introduced Cynthia to me. Among other things, they talked about each other's kids, and Carol put some smiles on Cyn's face. While she was in the hospital, Cyn kept asking me to turn up the oxygen level, although the machine, which was clipped on Cyn's finger, said that she was getting enough.

After leaving the hospital, Cynthia's physical condition hadn't improved much, but it seemed that her mind had cleared up a lot. I had talked with her doctor a few weeks before concerning the amount of morphine I should give her and the fact that I couldn't get her to eat hardly anything. I didn't ask him point blank about how many weeks or months did he think she had to live. I just said that it was clear to me that she was in the hands of the Lord, and he sort of acknowledged that it was the case. Of course, Cyn and I believed that it was in the hands of the Lord from the beginning. But we knew that the Lord also worked through the skills he had given to man and the doctors.

Cyn was steadily complaining about not getting enough oxygen, so Jason and I brought over the other oxygen concentrator machine from her mama's apartment. She could breathe better with both of them in her nose. I knew that they had said to give her a certain amount, but this was late in the game. I just couldn't refuse her. I called my cousin, Mason, who ran an oxygen concentrator business in Enterprise, Alabama. He gave me some pointers about how patients on oxygen think. But neither one of us knew that one of her lungs was practically gone, and the other was heavily damaged.

The doctor hinted that the insurance companies get sort of wary of paying continued hospitalization for terminally ill patients, but I didn't want to be alone in the house with Cyn while she fought for her last breath. Because I could just feel things coming, I took off a week earlier before the schools' Christmas holidays were to start. Jason needed a rest, and I didn't want him to have to make a critical decision or witness his mother's last breaths.

On that Monday night I had been working hard. I pulled Cyn out of the bed to use the portable toilet, gave her a bath, and I had to keep adjusting her on the bed for comfort. I was back in the living room looking at television. She sensed I was working hard, and I guess I must have been looking tired. She called me to the room. She said, "Sit down."

I rubbed her head like I liked to do, and held my lips on her fine, soft hair getting me some good head sugah.

I was sitting on the side of the bed. "What now, Woman? I know. You just can't stand for me to be out of your sight, huh? OK ...yes to anything you want of me."

In a light, sweet whisper she said, "Baby... you're getting tired of me, aren't you?"

"What! You mean I'm looking tired. Maybe, but I can never get tired of waiting on my baby. Cyn, you know that. I can do this for years. God gave me the job of taking care of you. Do you remember in sickness and in health, for better or worse?"

She was looking me in my eyes, and in her sweet, sweet light voice she said, "It can get better."

"I know, sweetheart. God can do anything if it is His will. We'll just pray again that he grant us a miracle."

And we held hands and prayed.

That night when I was lying in my room, I kept hearing her sweet voice saying, "It can get better." And at that late hour, I knew that only God could save her. I was swept again into one of those melancholic moods full of sadness and love. She was so brave and so spirit-filled. Lying in the dark, I thought again about some words she would always use when we prayed in duet. She would ask the Lord to send his angels to protect her. So in my prayers on that sad night I asked the Lord over and over to send His angels, too.

At this time, before I would go to sleep in my bed, I would sleep in her bed every night. I would only leave after she had gone to sleep. I had both of the oxygen levels up all the way. I told her this was more than she had in the hospital and the machine said that enough oxygen was in her blood. She said again that she could hardly breathe. So I let her use one of the portables for a while, and that helped. As I lay in the bed with her that night, I was really close, right up under her. It was very late when I went to my room.

That morning, she didn't call me like she would most of the times. I was sort of dreading to look in the room, as I had felt on so many nights before. When I entered the room, I noticed she was panting real hard, even with all three tanks going. When I sat on the side of the bed, she said nothing. She was just staring at me and panting for breath. I knew it was time, so I called 911 again, and I called Jason. It was the fire department paramedics this time; they said they were going to the nearest hospital. They carried her to South Shore Hospital, which is a five-minute drive from our house.

They didn't have a single patient in the emergency room. They got started right away once they understood she was an insurance patient. I'm not saying they would have acted differently if she didn't have insurance, but it makes a difference. Jason and I waited around and they soon took her up to a room. The doctor on duty showed me the X-rays of her lungs. One looked to be gone and the other looked about half its normal size. I had to fill out the standard forms, and they asked me the standard questions about any extraordinary means in case of cardiac arrest. I told them, like I had told Northwestern, not to use any of those methods. They put her on this machine. I really had been blessed so far as sickness among close family members, because I didn't know what a respirator machine was. I looked on the side of the machine, and I wrote down the long name for it so I could tell her doctor when I called him the next day.

I did call her doctor the next day. I told him why I had called for the paramedics, and where she was located. When I said that she was on a respirator, he seemed annoyed saying, "Why won't they let her die in peace?"

All indications to me were that it was the time, and I was relieved that he had confirmed it for me. Cyn really liked her doctor; she had a lot of faith in him. I didn't really know him, but because of Cyn's reaction to him, I felt as though he was superior in dealing with the psychological needs of a cancer patient. Even though Cyn was not in Northwestern, he told me to have the doctor at South Shore contact him, and he would bring him up to date on her condition.

I was glad she was in South Shore Hospital because it was on the South Side. Her mother and other friends could easily come and say good-bye. Her mother wasn't able to make any visits to the Loop and Northwestern. Jason and I took her over to the hospital the very next day. We were able to take her over several times, and we could leave her there to sit with Cyn. Other friends could easily come over too, and they did.

I walked over most of the time, just so I could think about the situation while coming and going. She couldn't talk with the machine in her mouth, but she tried to. I gave her a pen to write down what she was trying to say. I couldn't understand any of her writing, so the night before she went into the hospital was really our last two-way conversation. I told her what hospital she was in, and she understood that. I was also able to pick up on when she wanted me to take her mother home. It was Wednesday when she was placed on the respirator; by Saturday her consciousness was gone. Her eyes would open occasionally, but I could get no other response from her. She was there for a week, crossing over the River Jordan the next Wednesday.

There is a satisfaction in one's soul whether you win or lose when you have done the best that you can do. I felt that I had, even though I really wanted it to come from Cynthia's mouth.

However, reflecting, I guess she did tell me that I had done all right. Through my loneliness I felt the peace of knowing that she was now in paradise and a lot of the sorrow I had felt for her, I began to feel for myself.

When I was at home by myself that Wednesday night, I was bone-tired. The concentrator machines now turned off left the house totally silent. All around the house were medicines and all of those things used to fight cancer. They were lying in silence like muskets, cannons, and swelled bodies on a Civil War battlefield. I had made up the bed in her room and straightened things up, even though I had felt she was not coming back. I didn't get much rest the week she was in South Shore. I had been so used to being on alert that I couldn't just turn it off. I thought that if I said the Lord's Prayer out loud that I would hear her voice in duet again. And I did hear her, but it was only in my head. In my prayers I thanked the Lord for allowing me to be happy for so many years. I thanked Him for all of the other blessings he had bestowed upon me and Cynthia. I tried to just give myself total peace about things, but that peace would come and go in the next few days.

I thought a lot about my playing the last role in our love affair. They say that the Lord will not place a burden upon you that you can't handle. As hard as it had been, I felt that the Word was right. We can all do what God has assigned us to do, and I was only doing what so many other people do on every single day. People giving more of themselves in taking care of their dearest loved ones, in their loved one's worst hours of need.

I thought back to my connection with the slave wet-nurse. Her pain and her heroics didn't just last over a period of months, but she had to adjust to a way of life that was full of constant pain and sorrow. Like her, and not like the proverbial man, I had done what I had to do. As a lover, I had to play an unfamiliar role that I didn't want to play. Cynthia was an independent woman, and she and I both were in roles we didn't want to be in. It was a very difficult last few weeks, but they were not without loving moments and sweetness. All of our many happy years and technicolor days together came down to these few sad and precious ones. Bittersweet days and nights when she was literally my baby… and I was her mammy.

Stay Winter Day

I've heard that far north at the
top of the world you never leave

the sun is always shining,

don't leave me now, stay winter day,
winter day don't let the dark night
    find me all alone,
embrace me in this winter when I'm
    not strong.

    Great light,
I know the sunset is very beautiful,
    she seduces all
of us with spectacular colors, but
her crimson is your blood and her
purple will drape your sarcophagus.

    Stay winter day,
let your precious light keep shining,
    not forever,
just while I hide from loneliness.
I don't know loneliness but I feel
it lurking, waiting to catch me

in this my darkest hour.

Sweet sunshiny light linger, reign,
    don't leave me
grieving alone in the black early
    morning,
Stay winter day… winter day stay!

Rainstorm Come for Me

I smell you in the heavy air,
see your face in ominous clouds;
you've overrun the far horizon,

rainstorm come for me.

        Not
timidly as in a spring shower,
a pitter-patter quiet and gentle,
        and
don't run saline down my face
washing me as if you were tears.

        Come with
lightning and rolling thunder
        from
the place where you were born,
        rumbling
howling, pouring in the wind

rainstorm come for me.

Rainstorm, I stand in waiting,
holding nothing to cover me;
        drench me
with baptismal water from the
        Sea of Galilee,
flood places of my loneliness,
        and wash me in the blood,

cleansing rain — come for me.

Love Decided to Stay

she was
body, soul, love, spirit
when her body had broken
and lay cold
her soul, spirit, and love
ascended and held
each other's hand as they
rose heavenwards floating
like Angels

soon love
stopped the ascenders and
they dangled like
sunbeans divinely glowing,
love gazed back at me sad
empty, alone,

but she looked very happy
because love and happiness
are one,
her eyes were moisten soft
her smile bright, angelic
for sure she
was thinking about her one
promise to me,

love hugged, kissed them
told her soul and spirit
to fly away

"I think I'm going to stay"

Night Before the Funeral

The night before the funeral, I was to go with Jason to view the body. He was late, and the funeral home was about to close, so I left without him. Jason was the one who told me that Cynthia had passed. He had been to the hospital and sat in the room crying before the body was moved. The nurses were waiting for me to come before the body would be moved. I don't know whether that is the standard practice or not. The majority of the nurses on that floor seem to have been Philippine-Americans. They were good at their jobs and very nice. Earlier in the week, I took over my picture album of Cynthia and me in the good old days just to acquaint them better with the person they were taking care of.

I decided to wait until the funeral home got the body ready for showing before I viewed it. I was never one for viewing bodies because I know that the soul was gone; this wasn't the person anymore. Still, I was drawn to go, especially this time. I was getting calls, so I put out the word that there would be no formal viewing of the body. Vicky Williams asked me to place the Bible she had given Cynthia, with Cyn's name on it, in the casket. So I had the Bible when I went to the funeral home. I called and told the attendant what I wanted to do. It was near closing time, and I think he was waiting for me before closing. I handed him the Bible; he went to a room close by and was out in a second. I really don't know whether I had definitely planned to view the body, because I always like to remember people as they were. Since I had already asked for a closed-casket funeral, I expected the body to be in the back somewhere out of sight. But the attendant was in and out so fast, I was still standing there. Then I made a verbal gaffe. I asked him, "Is she dressed?" instead of, "Is the body ready for showing?"

He said "Yes," and I slowly headed for the room. I wouldn't say that I was scared, but my heart was pounding on my chest. I guess it was the anxiety of never wanting to see what I was about to see. The battle with cancer was long in many ways, but also very short. I was thinking about the night I first saw her, and that night at the intercessory prayer meeting when she said she was going to live with Jesus.

Before the Casket

Anything… but this,
Anywhere… but here,
Any woman… but her.

My heart was pounding and I was breathing heavily; I had to stand there for a few seconds just to catch my breath. Cyn had on the same white linen suit she had gotten married in just sixteen months ago; a wave of anger swept over me. I was thinking "Damn! Look what this fucking disease has done to my baby." I don't know why I reacted that way; I knew how she looked. Her hair had started to come back from radiation, and somehow I expected her to look at rest. I expected her to look like the pretty lady that I stared at while she was sleeping peacefully. Instead, she looked like she was very angry and still fighting the cancer.

I was able to say a little something in a quiet whisper, "I'm so sorry, Baby."

I don't know why, but I partly blamed myself because I couldn't save her, and I was thinking that all of our praying had gone for nothing. But I quickly thought that this was God's will, and I should accept it. God didn't have to let me meet her at all. Nor let me love her, be loved by her, and be happy for all of those years. I wanted to apologize for being mad and cursing in my thoughts. I was thinking that Cyn was in Heaven, and she was also in this room in spirit. She was looking down on me, so I had to be nice. I whispered and it was curious, at least for me, "Tell Jesus I said hello."

After pausing for a little while, I was trying to think of something definitive to say, especially since I felt she was there listening. It was back to being just me and Cyn together; us alone in a room. I just whispered, "Thank you, Cyn… My Joy… sweet thang… thank you for coming into my life and making me so happy."

I started to just say goodbye and throw a kiss, but I remembered how my mama and our family never liked goodbyes. So I blew my kiss toward the ceiling and whispered again, "See ya, Sweetheart." And I turned and left.

That long night was not over. Later I would receive a strange, wonderful call and a wonderful message from another one of Cynthia's close girlfriends. You may recall my writing about Melba, a close college girlfriend of Cynthia's. Melba was living back home in Oklahoma City. She called me on that same night before the funeral about a couple of hours after I had returned from the funeral home. It was close to 11:00 P.M. when I answered the phone. She told me her name, and she went on to say a few things to make sure that I remembered her. I did instantly, even though I didn't recall talking to her on the telephone before. It's not possible to contact everybody, but somehow the news about a death gets around by word of mouth; the bad news even moves from state to state. Melba was talking on and on about various subjects. She mentioned that it had really been a long time since she and Cynthia had talked to each other. I saw her as sparring around for the right words, and not wanting to just come out and say what she had called me to say. Then, abruptly, she cut off the small talk, and she asked to speak to Cynthia.

I was stunned. I thought she was just making small talk before saying condolences. I couldn't give her an answer right away, because she kept talking. Sort of rambling, she kept on talking for a good while. That was good for me, because I was trying to think of a gentle way to tell her. I eventually started with, "You know, Cynthia became sick ten months ago."

I started from the beginning with Cynthia discovering the lump. As delicately as I could, I worked my way up to saying that Cyn fought a great fight, but didn't make it, and the funeral was actually tomorrow. I can hear her voice, even now, clearly saying "Cynthia is dead?" Her statement is so clear in my mind, because I never liked the word "dead," nor do I use it for the most part. I prefer using passed, crossed-over, or in heaven.

Before Melba and I finished talking, I sort of pieced together what had happened. We were victims of the same sad, didn't-want-to-believe-it type emotions. Joe, a college friend of hers and Cynthia's, had called her that same night with an unconfirmed report that Cynthia had passed. Joe lives in Chicago; the information was unconfirmed because I hadn't placed it in the paper. Instead of asking me something like that outright, Melba apparently wanted me to confirm it without her asking.

On this very sad night, Melba and I had a long conversation. She gave me a gift that moved me deeply. Here was a close girlfriend that Cyn had known since she was a teenager and a freshman in college. Melba knew other men in and out of Cyn's life, Cyn's boyfriends, and her first husband. Women share a lot of things with their close girlfriends, and these girlfriends make judgments about the men in their lives. I hoped I had fared well, and apparently I did. Melba told me things I had not heard before. She told me her viewpoint on why Cyn was attracted to me, and she told me about the happiness I had brought to Cynthia's life.

One of the ways that Hollywood has messed up America is by constantly showing dying in a way that dying very seldom happens, the famous death scenes; the long death-bed conversations where the dying gets to lucidly tie up loose ends with everybody before they go. The ones that are left have all of their questions answered, and they walk away with the peace of mind that all has been said. All is not said. I felt that many things were left unsaid. But listening to Melba, I was spellbound. Her perceptiveness into what I wanted to hear was amazing, and without me asking, she was answering all of my questions. I'm a natural skeptic as opposed to being highly spiritual, but I felt this strange, wonderful feeling that Cynthia was talking to me through her. Cyn was talking to me from the other side. Melba sounded so much like Cyn. She had the same voice intonation, the logical reasoning, and the way Cyn put sentences together. I'll always believe it was Cyn telling me things she wanted to say, but couldn't. It was with a sweetness, a clarity that morphine would not allow Cyn to do in the final days. I could only listen and feel good. I know I had given her all of me. I had done my best, and now I was hearing that my best had been good enough. I've always wanted a good woman, and the main way I know to bring that about is for me to be a good man. I was very grateful to hear again, and for the final analysis, that I had brought Cyn the happiness and the joy she had given to me. I had a different, a spiritual, and a loving peace of mind when I hung up the phone. On that sad night, I was very grateful again for meeting and knowing all of those wonderful girlfriends of Cynthia's.

Sweet Life, Sweet Unfairness

So loved, sweet, precious, yet
so cruel, uneven, remorseless,
life why are you so unfair?

What has anyone done to you
    but love you,
embraced and fought for you;
you're in liaison with pain
suffering, sickness, and famine.
    You depart at a
time when you are the sweetest.
I'm also your victim, though
still loving and wanting you but
you've taken love away from me
dragging brutally and painfully.

I begged for mercy and you were
    unmerciful;
you made me watch and watched
    me crying in the night.

Sweet life, sweet unfairness,

    there is
someone who's greater than you;
    who will defeat you
as you have defeated me and mine.

    Brief life, hard life,
I know His everlasting name and
I'll magnify and glorify His name.

The Last Key

It was the last act; the ritual had been played out. The living had buried the dead, and friends and acquaintances from both sides of the marriage had paid their respects. People scurried back into the warmth of their cars escaping the cold of this wind-swept day, December 29, 1993.

I had vowed to remain dignified throughout the service. I tried to remember what everybody says at this time, "Her troubles are over." The mind game, painful memories, and emptiness for me had just begun. I was sitting on the passenger side of the front seat of a black Cadillac limousine. Two of my brothers, William and Alonza, were sitting on the second seat. My son and step-son, Oronde and Jason, were sitting on the back seat. Minutes ago, we were all standing in front of the casket as it slowly descended into the earth. The grave-side service was mercifully short, and I had held back my tears for most of the day, but the moisture in my eyes had overflowed as the casket slowly moved down on what looked like giant rubber bands. The tears were gently running down my face, but I didn't cry aloud. I refused to do so in front of everybody.

We had been mostly quiet, but we were humorous at points on the long ride to the cemetery. When the Gamble brothers get together, there's always a little humor, even under the worst of circumstances. A dignified-looking gentleman walked up and lightly tapped on the window of the limousine before I opened the door. He had that mulatto look that many African-American funeral directors seem to have. I believe it's a custom passed down from slavery days. The mixture of Christianity and the remnants of indigenous African religions of the early slave funerals vanished, and the light-skinned, privileged blacks came to dominate the funeral business. Anyway, he was a man that knew his job. He talked in a hushed, professional tone while efficiently taking care of business. He began by explaining the contents of a black case. The name of his funeral home, Taylor, was written on it in gold Old English script. It held the guest registration book, copies of death certificates, thank-you cards, envelopes, an obituary done in plastic, and extra copies of the obituary. I signed for them; then he voiced religious expressions of sympathy for me and my family before he departed.

Our two family limos were the last cars to leave the grave site, but they didn't head for the church and the repast right away. The limos simply drove out of one gate to the other side of the road, and then through the main gate of Lincoln Cemetery. We stopped beside the business building; everyone was asked if they would they like to use the washroom facilities. My wife's mother was helped out of the limo. As we sat in the car, it was quiet. I was reflecting on the other events of the day, and I could see right across the road to the grave site. The workers had quickly moved in with a flat-bed truck and a small earth-mover tractor. The truck had a crane on the back, and I guess it had been used to lower the heavy vault into the ground. It swung around, and the men lowered the lid onto the vault. One worker threw the green imitation carpet that surrounds the hole onto the back of the truck. Then the men, using hand shovels, began to throw in dirt, filling up the hole. I imagine the tractor finished filling up the hole, leveled and smoothed off the mound of fresh dirt, but by then we were gone.

Perhaps for those cemetery workers it was another day's

work; another stranger put into the ground. Perhaps what looked like haste to me, was efficiency at doing their jobs. Maybe they had to hurry to another spot in the cemetery. But what was casual to them was soul shattering to me. In my mind, they were in the presence of a real special person… my baby, unforgettable and irreplaceable. They should have moved respectfully slower. Maybe even looked a little more solemn with that quiet dignity of the funeral director. These were my private thoughts which were probably unfair to the workers. They didn't know who it was, let alone love her with all one's heart as I do.

Lastly, the dignified gentleman from Taylor Funeral Home handed me something that I have waited until now to mention. Maybe because it was so surprising or unexpected. After explaining to me, one by one, the contents of the case, he presented to me a brown and silver metal key. He said it was the key to the casket. I didn't know there was such a thing, and what was I supposed to do with it?

On the next day when I reviewed the contents of the black case, holding that key in my hand elicited strange, mixed feelings. It was still sort of surprising to me to have received such a different memento. A flower pressed between the pages of a Bible would seem to be more of a traditional thing to have received. Perhaps a beautiful yellow rose; something that had lived and bloomed with spectacular beauty, and something having brought a great joy before its end. As time passed, the rose would become dry, stiffened, and faded. It would have faded as I hope my deep hurt will fade someday. But that metal key will keep past my lifetime. The key would show no indication of passing time that brings about healing. Still, it was the last key shared between us, and the sharing of keys, physically and emotionally, is one of the cornerstones of a loving relationship. I thought keys are one of the first signs of trust because they're usually shared with family members or a close friend. So when single people give up their keys in a relationship that may have started out casually, I believe it's definitely a growing feeling of intimacy and love. I hadn't dated Cynthia two years before I gave her the keys to my apartment. I knew I was breaking one of the cardinal rules of bachelorhood, an act which means giving up some of one's independence, committing, and sharing of space. My days as a bachelor were not officially ended by saying "I do" and signing papers; that was years away. But my totally free bachelor days were unofficially over. I knew I wanted to "keep that woman." I wanted her to share my space, share my life, and she did.

The city of Chicago has become like a giant movie set to me. I move around every day coming across various places where our lives played out. Many sweet scenes return to me in slow motion. I get to better understand her hold on me. I try to decipher her complexity, even though, for the most part, it was enough for me to love her, to have her, and not completely understand her.

One of my favorite spirituals that I play all the time is from "Spirituals in Concert" with Jessye Norman and Kathleen Battle. It's Kathleen Battle's rendition of "Oh, Glory." There's a line in it that says, "Oh, Glory! There is room enough in Paradise/ To have a home in Glory!"

I plan to see Cyn, my father, and all of my friends that have passed on. And I plan to have a home in Glory.

Today, I'm in this world of grieving; I'm in search of healing and greater spirituality. I'm also in the world of the lonely and in the pursuit of happiness. But the story of Cyn and me isn't over, because she'll always be existential in my head.

Existential

She was predestined to be with me,
some how, some way, some day.

I think I created her in a dream,
I had awakened and she was there.

She must have
been born deep in my id, created by
my sense of aesthetics and eroticism,

rose and
stepped out of my subconsciousness
quintessential female,
everything I ever wanted in a woman.

Our days were technicolor,

we were happy, laughing, and loving,
now, our world of touching, breathing,
and sweetness is gone,

but whether I'm awake or slumbering
she's existential in my head,
smiling, teasing, and throwing kisses,

it's a haunting,
affectionate, quintessence of love.

And we'll die on the same day

because I'll always love her and
she'll always be in my consciousness
living as long as I live.

It's The Woman in My Soul

When I feel a
summer night wind gust in my sandals,
washing my bare feet, cool on my legs
as if it were female hands spreading
moisturizing lotion,

it's not the wind that's bringing joy;
it's the memories of a Chicago beauty
in cool, gusty, Windy City breezes,
it's the woman in my soul.

When I watch the sun on its way to
work in the morning,
stepping out of the lake's horizon,
getting ready to strut across the sky

my joy
is in more than the marigold sunrise,
it's memories of the sun on her face,
it's the woman in my soul.

In the heart of the city,
in twilight, in the electric forest,
as the stylish lady walks swiftly by
the scent
of her cologne is scanty, lecherous,
lingering in the air licking my face

but my joy isn't
solely in its erogenous familiarity,
all of my joy is in memories of her,

she's still making me happy,
it's the woman in my soul.

Not Again!

I had awakened to pitch blackness.
I'm not afraid of the dark; it was
just startling like it is sometimes.

In the seconds before my eyes could
focus in the bits of light that was
always peeking from under the door,
or filtering around edges of blinds
there was always faint breathing,

a pheromonal scent of body lotion,
a warm body to snuggle up against,
smooth shoulders to place my lips,

there was aromatic hair to sniff,
breast, unconfined by a nightgown,
        and soft
jutting buttocks flush on my belly.

        It wasn't
just a woman, she was my baby,
my one and only, irreplaceable.

When my eyes were focused, my mind
clear, I murmured in a wistful moan,
God, no! No! Don't let it be true!

        But it was true,
she's gone, she's with the saints,
not again! not again! not again!
but it is again, ...and I am again,
        alone in the dark.